LOSE WEIGHT BY EATING
Detox Week

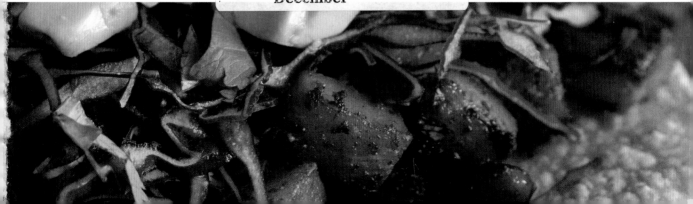

ALSO BY AUDREY JOHNS

LOSE WEIGHT BY EATING:

130 Amazing Clean-Eating Recipe Makeovers
for Guilt-Free Comfort Food

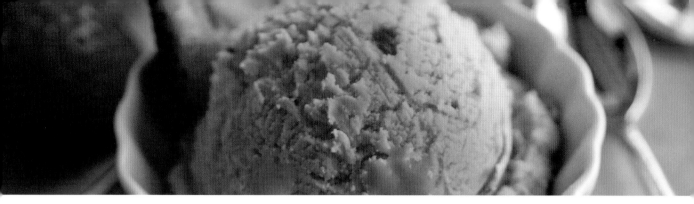

LOSE WEIGHT BY EATING
Detox Week

Twice the Weight Loss in Half the Time with 130 Recipes for a Crave-Worthy Cleanse

Audrey Johns

WM

WILLIAM MORROW

An Imprint of HarperCollinsPublishers

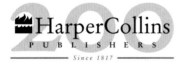

LOSE WEIGHT BY EATING: DETOX WEEK. Copyright © 2017 by Audrey Johns. All rights reserved. Printed in the United States of America. No part of this book may be used or reproduced in any manner whatsoever without written permission except in the case of brief quotations embodied in critical articles and reviews. For information address HarperCollins Publishers, 195 Broadway, New York, NY 10007.

HarperCollins books may be purchased for educational, business, or sales promotional use. For information please e-mail the Special Markets Department at SPsales@harpercollins.com.

FIRST EDITION

Designed by Paula Russell Szafranski
Photography by Carl Kravats

Library of Congress Cataloging-in-Publication Data has been applied for.

ISBN 978-0-06-266292-7

17 18 19 20 21 ID/QDG 10 9 8 7 6 5 4 3 2 1

For Kara—*my best friend, sister, soulmate, and support system.*

Thank you for thirty years of amazing friendship,

and cheers to another thirty. I adore you.

XOX

Contents

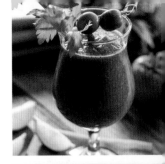

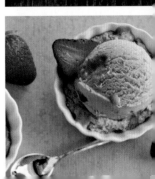

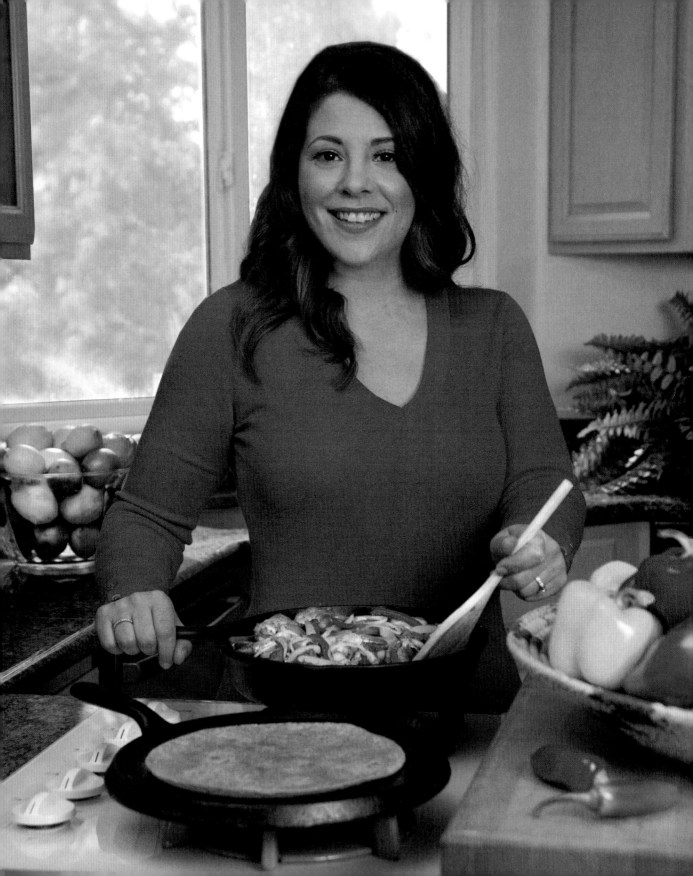

Introduction

I have struggled with my weight for my entire life. I was always the heaviest person in the room and people would say, "But she has such a pretty face." In 2011, I started my final weight-loss journey and by the following year I had lost 150 pounds in just eleven months. I documented my success and the tools I used to reach my goals on my blog, *Lose Weight by Eating*. Since then, I have kept the weight off . . . kind of.

I have fluctuated up and down 15 pounds over the years, partly because I'm a woman who experiences some monthly fluctuations and partly because I'm human and I make mistakes. After losing 150 pounds, 15 pounds is not a big deal, I agree, but on a woman who's a petite five foot three, it really shows! That's where the Detox Week comes into play. I use it to get back on track, to slim down fast for TV shows, and to reset my taste buds so I crave the healthy stuff.

Shortly after completing my first cookbook, *Lose Weight by Eating*, I created the original Detox Week. It quickly became the most popular page on my blog, and people started writing in to share that they had lost large amounts of weight, some up to 18 pounds in a single week! The most common requests were for a longer program and, of course, for more recipes.

Readers have used the programs to overcome plateaus, to jump-start weight loss, and to lose the last stubborn pounds they have been fighting for years. The exciting part is that after a single week on the program they start craving healthy food, so the usual weight regain after a short weight-loss program rarely happens. These Detox Week weight-loss superstars keep losing weight, simply because they don't crave fatty unhealthy food; they actually crave healthy foods.

Lose Weight by Eating has proven time and time again that it is what you eat that counts in weight loss, not how much you exercise, and these detox plans take that one step further with foods that will accelerate weight loss and raise your metabolism naturally. Yes, of course exercise is important for overall health and to help you tone up as you lose, but if you want to lose weight, you have to concentrate on what you eat and let your exercise take a backseat to your diet.

So what do I mean by *detox*? It means "to abstain from or rid the body of toxic or unhealthy substances," and in this book we will be abstaining from any food or drink that isn't natural, removing all toxic food from our diets and unhealthy substances from our drinks, and consuming ingredients that actually help rid the body of toxins and unhealthy substances. If you think of a detox as something really strict and harsh, just think of this as "detox lite"—a plan that's safe for all ages and stages of life.

- **We will abstain** from processed food and drinks that are filled with chemical-derived thickening agents, preservatives, fake sugars, and dyes.

- **We will *remove*** toxic food that is hurting both our weight-loss efforts and our overall health. Fried foods will be replaced with baked, sugars will be minimized, and unhealthy carbohydrates will be replaced with healthy versions.

- **We will *set aside*** the alcoholic beverages and unhealthy substances in our drinks and swap fake sugars for cleansing waters, but don't worry—we have mocktails and fancy drinks for you and your taste buds to enjoy!

- **We will fill** our diet with food and drinks that actually help rid the body of toxins!

We will not be fasting, taking any kind of diet pill, or adding any unnatural, pre-packaged foods or beverages to our diets. Those detox drinks, foods, pills, and products that weight-loss companies push are just a waste of your money—all you'll get is clever marketing and no lasting results. What will you need to buy on this detox plan? Just groceries!

So let's shake things up and reset our view on food. Think about it this way—if there's a commercial for a food product, there's a 95 percent chance that it is advertising junk food that is packed full of chemicals, preservatives, and sugar (or worse, fake sugar!). What's in the remaining 5 percent? Real foods, like milk or produce such as avocados and oranges (not mass-produced guacamole or orange juice—do you see the distinction?). If you can identify clever marketing, you can pinpoint mass-produced food and remove it from your diet and then replace it with foods from farms, not huge factories.

That leads us to a good rule of thumb: If it doesn't have a label, it's most likely a good choice. Think less about convenience and more about how the food will affect your body. Sure, you might have to look up the calories for an apple, but that fruit boosts your metabolism and its fiber scrubs your insides clean and keeps you full, while that 100-calorie bag of "snacks" is packed full of not just chemicals and preservatives that tell your body to hold on to fat but also overprocessed, even fake, sugar that causes weight gain. An apple—label-free—is the healthy choice; your body knows how to process it. Remember, we are animals and we need to eat from nature, not from a laboratory!

Now let's talk about food quality. I know that many of you won't be able to purchase organic food, whether for cost or access reasons, and that's fine . . . but if you can, organic is always best! You don't want to remove all those chemicals from processed foods just to replace them with pesticides, so at the very least, look at the price difference and weigh where you can afford organic and where you cannot. Many people do the detox plan without purchasing organic and then love it so much and feel so great eating healthy that they take the next step and go organic. My hope is that eventually everyone can afford to go all organic, but until then, you have to do what you feel is best for you and your family. You have my opinion—now it's time for you to formulate yours.

Let's dig into the program!

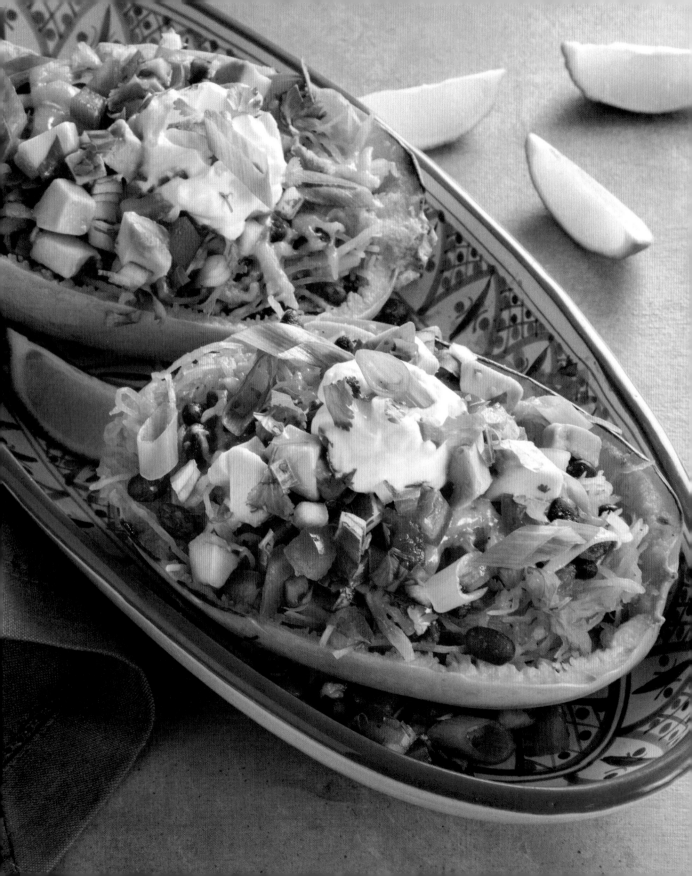

1

The Customizable Lose Weight by Eating Detox Plans

Welcome to your customized detox plan! We have four plans here for you to choose from, and best of all, they work together, so you can flow from one to the other as your needs change. Start by taking the fifteen-question Detox Quiz below, or go ahead and read over the four plans that follow and choose the one you feel is best for you.

Don't start with the hardest plan—if you love the ease of the one-week plan and want to keep going or start the three-month plan, go for it, but start out with baby steps so it won't be so daunting.

Detox Quiz! 15 Questions Get You a Customized Detox Plan

Yes, you can go ahead and write in this book . . . but I prefer to fill out the answers on removable Post-it notes—this way, should I pass on the book to a friend, I'm not airing out all my business, too. ;)

Are you pregnant or a nursing mom? If you are, skip the quiz and go to The Detox Lifestyle (page 15), which outlines a plan that is safe for pregnant women and nursing moms.

1. **How much weight do you want to lose?**
   a. 10 to 15 pounds
   b. 15 to 25 pounds
   c. 25 to 30+ pounds
   d. I'm not looking to lose much, maybe 5 to 10 pounds

2. **How old are you?**
   a. 25 to 45
   b. 18 to 25
   c. 45 to 60
   d. 60+

3. **What diets have worked for you in the past?**
   a. Short 1-week programs
   b. 30-day boot camps
   c. Meal-planning services
   d. Long-term group plans

4. **How often do you exercise?**
   a. 2+ hours per week
   b. Once a week
   c. 5+ hours per week
   d. Monthly or less

5. **How quickly do you want to lose weight?**
   a. 7 days
   b. 30 days
   c. 3 months
   d. 6+ months

6. **Do you prefer to lose weight quickly or slowly?**
   a. Quickly
   b. Slowly
   c. I don't know
   d. Happy with my weight; just looking for healthier food choices

7. **Do you have an event you want to lose weight for? When is this event?**
   a. 1 to 2 weeks
   b. 4 weeks
   c. 3+ months
   d. Nope, no event coming up

8. **How much time do you spend cooking per day?**
   a. 10 to 15 minutes
   b. 30 minutes
   c. 1 hour
   d. More than 1 hour

9. **How often do you go out to eat?**
   a. Daily
   b. Once a week
   c. 2+ times per week
   d. Monthly

10. **How often do you snack?**
   a. All day, help!
   b. 2 to 3 times a day
   c. Not a snacker
   d. I get to snack and lose weight? Yippee!

11. How do you feel about green smoothies?

   a. Yum, love them!

   b. Willing to try

   c. Not so sure

   d. Eww . . . yuck!

12. How often do you eat veggies?

   a. Once a day

   b. Once in a while

   c. Almost never

   d. 2 to 3 times a day

13. How many calories do you eat per day?

   a. Fewer than 1,400

   b. 1,500 to 1,700

   c. More than 1,700

   d. No clue!

14. What's your favorite food group?

   a. Drive-thru!

   b. Sweets

   c. Carbs

   d. Veggies and fruit, yum!

15. How would you characterize your eating habits?

   a. Whatever's fast and easy

   b. Sometimes healthy, sometimes not . . .

   c. I love to cook at home

   d. Pretty darn healthy, if I do say so myself!

ANSWER KEY

MOSTLY A: Try out the Detox Week. This plan will help reset your taste buds to enjoy healthy food, and the program has lots of quick meals so you won't be tempted to go through a drive-thru. You'll most likely want to continue after the seven-day program, and I recommend the Detox Month if you want to keep going after Detox Week.

MOSTLY B: Try the Detox Month; it's easy to follow and filled with yummy food. The program will boost your metabolism and retrain your taste buds to enjoy vegetables.

MOSTLY C: I think you would love the 3-Month Detox Plan! After the three months are up, you'll feel so great you'll want to keep going with the Detox Lifestyle.

MOSTLY D: Start on the Detox Lifestyle, and if after a week or two you're looking for something more aggressive, add in a Detox Week once a month to boost weight loss.

THE FOUR DETOX PLANS, IN BRIEF

Detox Week	**3-Month Detox Plan**
see below	page 11
Detox Month	**Detox Lifestyle**
page 9	(365 days, plan safe enough for pregnant and nursing moms), page 15

Detox Week

The original is always the best place to start! My blog readers lose on average 10 pounds on this seven-day plan.

WHAT TO EAT:

Detox Week

Day 1	*1 smoothie (chapters 2–3)*	*1 salad (chapters 4–7)*	*1 meal* (chapters 8–12)*	*2 snacks (chapters 14–15)*
Day 2	*1 smoothie (chapters 2–3)*	*1 salad (chapters 4–7)*	*1 salad (chapters 4–7)*	*2 snacks (chapters 14–15)*
Day 3	*1 smoothie (chapters 2–3)*	*1 salad (chapters 4–7)*	*1 smoothie (chapters 2–3)*	*2 snacks (chapters 14–15)*
Day 4	*1 smoothie (chapters 2–3)*	*1 smoothie (chapters 2–3)*	*1 smoothie (chapters 2–3)*	*2 snacks (chapters 14–15)*
Day 5	*1 smoothie (chapters 2–3)*	*1 smoothie (chapters 2–3)*	*1 smoothie (chapters 2–3)*	*2 snacks (chapters 14–15)*
Day 6	*1 smoothie (chapters 2–3)*	*1 salad (chapters 4–7)*	*1 salad (chapters 4–7)*	*2 snacks (chapters 14–15)*
Day 7	*1 smoothie (chapters 2–3)*	*1 salad (chapters 4–7)*	*1 meal* (chapters 8–12)*	*2 snacks (chapters 14–15)*

*Or you can use any recipe from the original *Lose Weight by Eating* cookbook or from the website as a meal on days 1 and 7.

WHAT TO DRINK:

DAILY: 1 gallon of water throughout the day and 1 cup of tea or coffee (see Tips for Keeping Coffee and Tea All Natural on page 248)
WEEKLY: 3 drinks from chapter 13
EXERCISE: 3 hours of exercise for the week
REST: 8 to 9 hours of sleep per night

KEEP GOING:

Often by day 5, people ask, "Can I just keep going after day 7?" If you are one of these readers, you can easily transition into the Detox Month or the 3-Month Detox Plan, as both plans begin with a Detox Week! If you've lost all the weight you're looking to lose and just want to maintain, the Detox Lifestyle is your best choice to maintain your weight loss.

Detox Month

The Detox Month is great if you want to get rid of the last 10 to 25 pounds you've been trying to lose for years, look great for an upcoming trip, or simply reset your taste buds, all on a thirty-day plan.

WHAT TO EAT:

WEEK 1: Detox Week (see the menu plan opposite)
WEEK 2: Modified Detox Week (see the menu plan on page 10)
WEEK 3: Detox Week
WEEK 4: Modified Detox Week

Most people like to have their smoothie at breakfast, salad at lunch, and meal at dinner, but you can mix these up however you like. Just note these changes when you fill out your Weekly Food Log (page 21).

Modified Detox Week

Day 1	1 smoothie (chapters 2–3)	1 salad (chapters 4–7)	1 meal* (chapters 8–12)	2 snacks (chapters 14–15)
Day 2	1 smoothie (chapters 2–3)	1 salad (chapters 4–7)	1 meal* (chapters 8–12)	2 snacks (chapters 14–15)
Day 3	1 smoothie (chapters 2–3)	1 salad (chapters 4–7)	1 meal* (chapters 8–12)	2 snacks (chapters 14–15)
Day 4	1 smoothie (chapters 2–3)	1 salad (chapters 4–7)	1 meal* (chapters 8–12)	2 snacks (chapters 14–15)
Day 5	1 smoothie (chapters 2–3)	1 salad (chapters 4–7)	1 meal* (chapters 8–12)	2 snacks (chapters 14–15)
Day 6	1 smoothie (chapters 2–3)	1 salad (chapters 4–7)	1 meal* (chapters 8–12)	2 snacks (chapters 14–15)
Day 7	1 smoothie (chapters 2–3)	1 salad (chapters 4–7)	1 meal* (chapters 8–12)	2 snacks (chapters 14–15)

*Or you can use any recipe from the original *Lose Weight by Eating* cookbook or from the website as a meal.

WHAT TO DRINK:

DAILY: 1 gallon of water throughout the day and 1 cup of tea or coffee (see Tips for Keeping Coffee and Tea All Natural on page 248)
WEEKLY: 3 drinks from chapter 13
EXERCISE: 3 hours of exercise for the week on weeks 1 and 2; 4 hours for weeks 3 and 4.
REST: 8 to 9 hours of sleep per night

KEEP GOING:

If you love the Detox Month, you can start the 3-Month Detox Plan or go right into the Detox Lifestyle; both plans will help you continue to lose weight while feeling great! You can also do another Detox Month if you prefer.

The 3-Month Detox Plan

This plan is a great way to drop weight fast, the natural way! You can expect to lose up to 50 pounds in three months. This plan is great if you want to use recipes from this book as well as the first *Lose Weight by Eating* cookbook.

WHAT TO EAT:

WEEK 1: Traditional Detox Week

WEEK 2: Traditional Detox Week, with an extra all-smoothie day

WEEK 3: Modified Detox Week, plus 1 free day

WEEK 4: Traditional Detox Week

WEEK 5: Traditional Detox Week, with an extra all-smoothie day

WEEK 6: Modified Detox Week, plus 1 free day

WEEK 7: Traditional Detox Week

WEEK 8: Traditional Detox Week, with an extra all-smoothie day

WEEK 9: Modified Detox Week, plus 1 free day

WEEK 10: Traditional Detox Week

WEEK 11: Traditional Detox Week, with an extra all-smoothie day

WEEK 12: Modified Detox Week, plus 1 free day

Detox Month

WEEK 1	1 smoothie
	1 salad
	1 detox
	  meal
	2 snacks
		1 smoothie
		2 salads
		2 snacks
			2 smoothies
			1 salad
			2 snacks
				3 smoothies
				2 snacks
					3 smoothies
					2 snacks
						1 smoothie
						2 salads
						2 snacks
							1 smoothie
							1 salad
							1 detox
							  meal
							2 snacks

WEEK 2	1 smoothie
	1 salad
	1 detox
	  meal
	2 snacks
		1 smoothie
		2 salads
		2 snacks
			3 smoothies
			2 snacks
				3 smoothies
				2 snacks
					3 smoothies
					2 snacks
						1 smoothie
						2 salads
						2 snacks
							1 smoothie
							1 salad
							1 detox
							  meal
							2 snacks

WEEK 3	1 smoothie
	1 salad
	1 detox
	  meal
	2 snacks
		1 smoothie
		2 salads
		2 snacks
			2 smoothies
			1 salad
			2 snacks
				FREE DAY!	3 smoothies
					2 snacks
						1 smoothie
						2 salads
						2 snacks
							1 smoothie
							1 salad
							1 detox
							  meal
							2 snacks

WEEK 4	1 smoothie
	1 salad
	1 detox
	  meal
	2 snacks
		1 smoothie
		2 salads
		2 snacks
			2 smoothies
			1 salad
			2 snacks
				3 smoothies
				2 snacks
					3 smoothies
					2 snacks
						1 smoothie
						2 salads
						2 snacks
							1 smoothie
							1 salad
							1 detox
							  meal
							2 snacks

WEEK 5	1 smoothie
	1 salad
	1 detox
	  meal
	2 snacks
		1 smoothie
		2 salads
		2 snacks
			2 smoothies
			1 salad
			2 snacks
				3 smoothies
				2 snacks
					3 smoothies
					2 snacks
						1 smoothie
						2 salads
						2 snacks
							1 smoothie
							1 salad
							1 detox
							  meal
							2 snacks

WEEK 6	1 smoothie
	1 salad
	1 detox
	  meal
	2 snacks
		1 smoothie
		2 salads
		2 snacks
			2 smoothies
			1 salad
			2 snacks
				FREE DAY!	3 smoothies
					2 snacks
						1 smoothie
						2 salads
						2 snacks
							1 smoothie
							1 salad
							1 detox
							  meal
							2 snacks

WEEK 7	1 smoothie 1 salad 1 detox meal 2 snacks	1 smoothie 2 salads 2 snacks	2 smoothies 1 salad 2 snacks	3 smoothies 2 snacks	3 smoothies 2 snacks	1 smoothie 2 salads 2 snacks	1 smoothie 1 salad 1 detox meal 2 snacks
WEEK 8	1 smoothie 1 salad 1 detox meal 2 snacks	1 smoothie 2 salads 2 snacks	3 smoothies 2 snacks	3 smoothies 2 snacks	3 smoothies 2 snacks	1 smoothie 2 salads 2 snacks	1 smoothie 1 salad 1 detox meal 2 snacks
WEEK 9	1 smoothie 1 salad 1 detox meal 2 snacks	1 smoothie 2 salads 2 snacks	2 smoothies 1 salad 2 snacks	FREE DAY!	3 smoothies 2 snacks	1 smoothie 2 salads 2 snacks	1 smoothie 1 salad 1 detox meal 2 snacks
WEEK 10	1 smoothie 1 salad 1 detox meal 2 snacks	1 smoothie 2 salads 2 snacks	2 smoothies 1 salad 2 snacks	3 smoothies 2 snacks	3 smoothies 2 snacks	1 smoothie 2 salads 2 snacks	1 smoothie 1 salad 1 detox meal 2 snacks
WEEK 11	1 smoothie 1 salad 1 detox meal 2 snacks	1 smoothie 2 salads 2 snacks	3 smoothies 2 snacks	3 smoothies 2 snacks	3 smoothies 2 snacks	1 smoothie 2 salads 2 snacks	1 smoothie 1 salad 1 detox meal 2 snacks
WEEK 12	1 smoothie 1 salad 1 detox meal 2 snacks	1 smoothie 2 salads 2 snacks	2 smoothies 1 salad 2 snacks	FREE DAY!	3 smoothies 2 snacks	1 smoothie 2 salads 2 snacks	1 smoothie 1 salad 1 detox meal 2 snacks

A note about your **FREE DAY:** This is not an open invitation to blow the entire diet! You will still need to stick to the key detox plan guidelines that have already been addressed: no fake food, no fried food, and certainly no fast food. But get your favorite meal at your favorite restaurant or make your favorite family meal; if your birthday is this week, enjoy a slice of cake (just one!), and if you're going out, get that glass of wine you've been yearning for (one glass of wine is okay, but no sugary cocktails and I'm sorry to say, stay away from the beer—it will only cause bloating).

You can take your free day any day of the week in which it falls—just choose the day you want.

Want an example of a healthy free day? Here's my ideal free day:

BREAKFAST: Strawberry Pancakes (page 217)
LUNCH: 3 street tacos from my favorite restaurant plus a few chips with unlimited salsa
DINNER: Vegetarian Lasagna (page 152)
SNACKS: Mini Pumpkin Spice Scones with Chocolate Pecan Glaze (page 270) and Hot Spinach Cheese Dip with Veggie Sticks (page 284)
DRINKS: 1 gallon of water and 1 glass of Chardonnay

WHAT TO DRINK:

DAILY: 1 gallon of water throughout the day and 1 cup of tea or coffee (see Tips for Keeping Coffee and Tea All Natural on page 248)
WEEKLY: 3 drinks from chapter 13
EXERCISE: 3 hours of exercise for the week on weeks 1 and 2; 4 hours on weeks 3 through 7; and 5 hours on weeks 8 through 12
REST: 8 to 9 hours of sleep per night

KEEP GOING:

If you want to continue after the 3-Month Detox Plan is over and you have more weight to lose, I recommend either a Detox Month or another 3-Month Detox Plan, depending on how much you have to lose. It would be beneficial to retake the quiz on page 6 if you are unsure. You can also go right into the Detox Lifestyle; it will help you continue to lose weight while feeling great. If you lost all the weight you are looking to lose, the Detox Lifestyle will also help you maintain your weight loss.

The Detox Lifestyle

Readers can expect to lose up to 15 pounds per month on this plan, and it's also a great way to maintain your current weight after weight loss. It's called a lifestyle, as it is not a time-limited weight-loss program, which is always the ideal way to lose weight. If you feel the other programs are too extreme for you, start here and do a Detox Week after a month or two, when you feel comfortable with the food and want to accelerate weight loss.

This plan is ideal for all ages and all stages of life. If you're pregnant or a nursing mom, this is safe enough for you and the little bundle of joy you're nourishing, with one modification: When the menu calls for a meal to be a smoothie, pregnant women and nursing moms should enjoy the smoothie alongside a healthy meal from chapters 4 through 12. Also, start out as outlined below; should you find yourself more hungry, add an extra snack.

WHAT TO EAT:

In this plan you will choose a breakfast, lunch, and dinner from the following chapters or from my first cookbook, *Lose Weight by Eating.* You'll need to swap four meals a week for smoothies (pregnant and nursing moms will enjoy a smoothie with a light meal) and have five salads per week as meals. Here's how you set up a menu for the week on this plan:

STEP 1: Flip to page 16 for a menu planner, or print one from my website (www.loseweightbyeating.com).

STEP 2: Choose one or two smoothies from chapter 2 or 3 and add them to four meal slots on the menu; for the smoothies and salads, I like to choose one or two recipes and alternate them on the menu.

STEP 3: Choose one to three salads from chapters 4 through 7 and add them to five meal slots on the menu.

STEP 4: Fill in the rest of the meal slots with recipes from this book and the original *Lose Weight by Eating* cookbook. I like to choose just one or two breakfast and lunch recipes and alternate them, to save money and to use leftovers better.

STEP 5: Choose a few snacks from chapters 14 and 15 and fill in the snack areas.

STEP 6: Place the week's menu in your planner or on your fridge for easy referencing.

Here is an example of a full week:

	BREAKFAST	LUNCH	DINNER	SNACK
MONDAY	Blueberry Apple Pie Smoothie (page 33)	Butternut Squash Chili (page 117)	Chinese Chicken Salad (page 88)	French Onion Dip with Veggie Sticks (page 277) and Watermelon Ice Pop (page 266)
TUESDAY	Grown-Up Strawberry Banana Smoothie (page 30)	Summer Salad with Nectarines and Avocado (page 70)	Surf-and-Turf Fajitas (page 164)	Strawberry Banana Bonbons (page 253) and Homemade Hummus with Veggie Sticks (page 287)
WEDNESDAY	Blueberry Apple Pie Smoothie (page 33)	Butternut Squash Chili (page 117)	Green Goddess Salad Wrap (page 99)	Rainbow Fruit Salad (page 257) and Pita Pizza Triangles (page 285)
THURSDAY	Grown-Up Strawberry Banana Smoothie (page 30)	Chinese Chicken Salad (page 88)	Skinny Chicken Parmesan with Roasted Broccoli (page 173)	French Onion Dip with Veggie Sticks (page 277) and Watermelon Ice Pop (page 266)
FRIDAY	Lemon Cranberry Breakfast Quinoa (page 213)	Summer Salad with Nectarines and Avocado (page 70)	Teriyaki Turkey Burgers with Potato Salad (page 204)	Strawberry Banana Bonbons (page 253) and Homemade Hummus with Veggie Sticks (page 287)
SATURDAY	Breakfast Tacos (page 224)	Chicken, Rice, and Black Bean Burrito Bowl (page 148)	Easy Chicken Cordon Bleu with French Bistro Salad (page 195)	Rainbow Fruit Salad (page 257) and Pita Pizza Triangles (page 285)
SUNDAY	Strawberry Pancakes (page 217)	Ceviche Tostadas (page 139)	Slow Cooker "Chunky" Beef Stew (page 146)	French Onion Dip with Veggie Sticks (page 277) and Watermelon Ice Pop (page 266)

Here is an example of a full week for pregnant women and nursing moms:

	BREAKFAST	LUNCH	DINNER	SNACK
MONDAY	Blueberry Apple Pie Smoothie (page 33) and Strawberry Pancakes (page 217)	Butternut Squash Chili (page 117)	Chinese Chicken Salad (page 88)	French Onion Dip with Veggie Sticks (page 277) and Watermelon Ice Pop (page 266)
TUESDAY	Grown-Up Strawberry Banana Smoothie (page 30) and Lemon Cranberry Breakfast Quinoa (page 213)	Summer Salad with Nectarines and Avocado (page 70)	Surf-and-Turf Fajitas (page 164)	Strawberry Banana Bonbons (page 253) and Homemade Hummus with Veggie Sticks (page 287)
WEDNESDAY	Blueberry Apple Pie Smoothie (page 33) and Strawberry Pancakes (page 217)	Butternut Squash Chili (page 117)	Green Goddess Salad Wrap (page 99)	Rainbow Fruit Salad (page 257) and Pita Pizza Triangles (page 285)
THURSDAY	Grown-Up Strawberry Banana Smoothie (page 30) and Lemon Cranberry Breakfast Quinoa (page 213)	Chinese Chicken Salad (page 88)	Skinny Chicken Parmesan with Roasted Broccoli (page 173)	French Onion Dip with Veggie Sticks (page 277) and Watermelon Ice Pop (page 266)
FRIDAY	Blueberry Apple Pie Smoothie (page 33) and Strawberry Pancakes (page 217)	Summer Salad with Nectarines and Avocado (page 70)	Teriyaki Turkey Burgers with Potato Salad (page 204)	Strawberry Banana Bonbons (page 253) and Homemade Hummus with Veggie Sticks (page 287)
SATURDAY	Breakfast Tacos (page 224)	Chicken, Rice, and Black Bean Burrito Bowl (page 148)	Easy Chicken Cordon Bleu with French Bistro Salad (page 195)	Rainbow Fruit Salad (page 257) and Pita Pizza Triangles (page 285)
SUNDAY	Strawberry Pancakes (page 217)	Ceviche Tostadas (page 139)	Slow Cooker "Chunky" Beef Stew (page 146)	French Onion Dip with Veggie Sticks (page 277) and Watermelon Ice Pop (page 266)

WHAT TO DRINK:

DAILY: 1 gallon of water throughout the day and 1 cup of tea or coffee (see Tips for Keeping Coffee and Tea All Natural on page 248)
WEEKLY: 3 drinks from chapter 13
EXERCISE: 3 hours of exercise per week for the first month; 4 hours per week month 2; 5 hours per week for month 3, and so on
REST: 8 to 9 hours of sleep per night

KEEP GOING:

This plan is a lifestyle, not a diet—and trust me, once you've enjoyed a full month on this plan, you'll feel so amazing that you'll want to keep it up.

If you hit a plateau or want to boost weight loss, try one of the shorter plans (the Detox Week or Detox Month) to increase your metabolism.

Overall Health for All!

Now, what if you already have a weight-loss plan you love, or what if you don't have any weight to lose? If you choose to skip over the weight-loss programs altogether and go straight to cooking the recipes, you'll still find great value in this book.

When my cookbook *Lose Weight by Eating* first came out, I had two different people from two different areas in the United States inform me that all the people in their local Weight Watchers groups were cooking from the book, as the recipes worked for both the *Lose Weight by Eating* program and Weight Watchers program. I love that people found ways to work the cookbook into the weight-loss programs they were already enjoying, and so in that same spirit these recipes and tips will help you in your journey, no matter what path you're on. To help you out, I added nutritional information to all the recipes in this book.

Even if you're not looking to lose weight, these recipes will fill your body with loads of nutrition. You'll notice that your skin will clear up, and your tummy troubles will ease. You'll have much more energy and may even start on the path of living longer. And all the recipes are safe for kids. We're not skimping on food here: When you have a smoothie you are eating the equivalent of 1½ salads, and we all know how healthy and nutrition-packed fresh salads are. So if your child asks for a sip of your smoothie and then drinks half of it (the way mine does), next time make extra and give her one of her own. You can feel good knowing you're instilling healthy habits now that will benefit your child for a lifetime.

Comparing the Two
Lose Weight by Eating Books

How is this book different from the original Lose Weight by Eating plan? If you love the original plan, you'll really love this one. If the first book was elementary school, this one is middle school. While these recipes are very accessible, I introduce some of the most popular superfoods, and a few ingredients might be new to you. But don't worry—the recipes are just as delicious, and we're simply visiting the health food store, not moving in altogether. You can still use the original Lose Weight by Eating plan with these recipes, maybe throwing in a Detox Week before a vacation (or after, if you eat too much naughty stuff), and of course you can start on the Detox Lifestyle and use recipes from both cookbooks to further continue your "education."

How Else Can I Use This Book?

This book is great for both short bursts and long-haul weight-loss and detox needs. You can use these recipes with any weight-loss plan and revisit the Detox Week and other plans outlined in this chapter to do all the following:

- Jump-start weight loss.

- Overcome plateaus.

- Reset your system after a (food- or alcohol-related) hangover.

- Retrain your taste buds and body to crave healthy food.

The Detox Week has proven time and time again that it can help readers jump-start their weight loss—often readers lose over 15 pounds in a single week. If you've hit a plateau, the Detox Month can help you get over that hump and get you back on the highway to weight loss. If you've eaten or drunk too much, choose to do a Detox Week, or even just a single day on the Detox Week to help reset your body and get you on the road to feeling better. Finally, all these programs help reset your taste buds so that you will actually start craving healthy foods. After just a week on the program, you'll actually crave salads!

Weight-Loss Log

Every little bit adds up. Don't be discouraged by a low weight-loss week—next week will be better! A 2.5-pound weight loss per week equals 130 pounds in a year. Remember, slow and steady wins the race.

DATE	NUMBER OF POUNDS LOST OR GAINED

Total # of pounds lost: _____ ÷ 8 = _____ (total eight-week average)

Weekly Food Log

	MONDAY	TUESDAY	WEDNESDAY	THURSDAY	FRIDAY	SATURDAY	SUNDAY
WATER							
BREAKFAST							
LUNCH							
DINNER							
SNACKS							
TOTAL CALORIES							

2

Delicious Detox Smoothies

Green smoothies are a great way to increase your veggie intake without actually tasting the veggies! Once you blend these veggies with yummy, naturally sweet fruits, all you taste is the fruit, making these great for all ages. My daughter loves green smoothies, and yes, they're part of the detox plans, but they are also full, healthy meals, so all ages can enjoy them! Pregnant women and nursing moms are good to go with these recipes, too. (See page 15 for more meal instructions.)

You can use fresh or frozen fruit in all these recipes. Often a recipe will call for frozen fruit; this is to help thicken the consistency and keep the smoothie cold, but you can swap fresh for frozen or frozen for fresh depending on what's available and your personal preference.

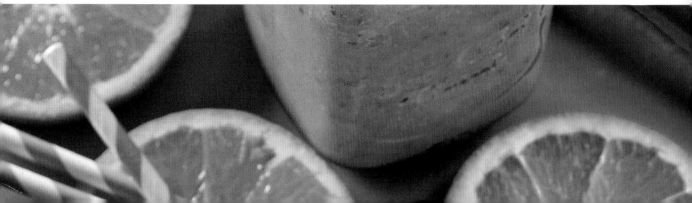

Sunrise Smoothie

When I first made this smoothie, my daughter, Sophia, drank almost all of it, leaving me with just a few sips, so the next time I increased the amount, to make enough for her and me, and she again finished all of hers and most of mine. These are kid-approved (or in my case, kid-demanded) mostly because of the taste but also because it's fun to swirl the colors.

Makes 2 servings | *Serving size: 8 to 10 ounces (depending on how thin you like it)*
Per serving: calories 144; fat 3 g; saturated fat 2 g; fiber 5 g; protein 2 g;
carbohydrates 31 g; sugar 23 g | *Prep time: 15 minutes* | *Cook time: 0 minutes*

YELLOW LAYER
1 banana
¼ cup frozen pineapple chunks
1 tablespoon unsweetened coconut flakes

PINK LAYER
½ cup frozen strawberries
¼ cup frozen peach slices

ORANGE LAYER
1 orange, peeled and segmented
¼ cup frozen mango chunks

1. Place all the yellow layer ingredients in a blender, add ¼ cup water, and blend until smooth, adding more water 2 tablespoons at a time as needed to thin it. You want it thick, so add just enough water to help it blend. Higher-quality blenders will need less water than lower-quality blenders. Divide the yellow layer between two glasses. Do not wash out the blender.

2. Place the pink layer ingredients in the blender, add ¼ cup water, and blend until smooth, adding more water 2 tablespoons at a time as needed to thin it. Keep the consistency the same as the yellow layer. Spoon the pink layer on top of the yellow layer in both glasses. Do not wash out the blender.

3. Place the orange layer ingredients in the blender, add ¼ cup water, and blend until smooth, adding more water 2 tablespoons at a time as needed to thin it. Keep the consistency the same as the yellow and pink layers. Gently spoon some on top of the pink layer (this will keep it from sinking to the bottom) in both glasses, then gently divide the rest of the orange layer between the two glasses. Some of the layers will automatically spill into each other, but don't stress—they're meant to taste delicious together. This is why you don't wash out the blender after each layer, so the flavors all marry a little . . . and to save you some time, too.

VARIATIONS
- Make it a green smoothie! Add 1 grated carrot to the orange layer and ½ cup spinach to the pink layer. The spinach will change the color a little but you won't be able to taste it, and the carrot will only make the bottom layer more vibrant.
- Up the protein! Adding ⅓ cup Greek yogurt to each layer adds 24 grams of protein to each shake.

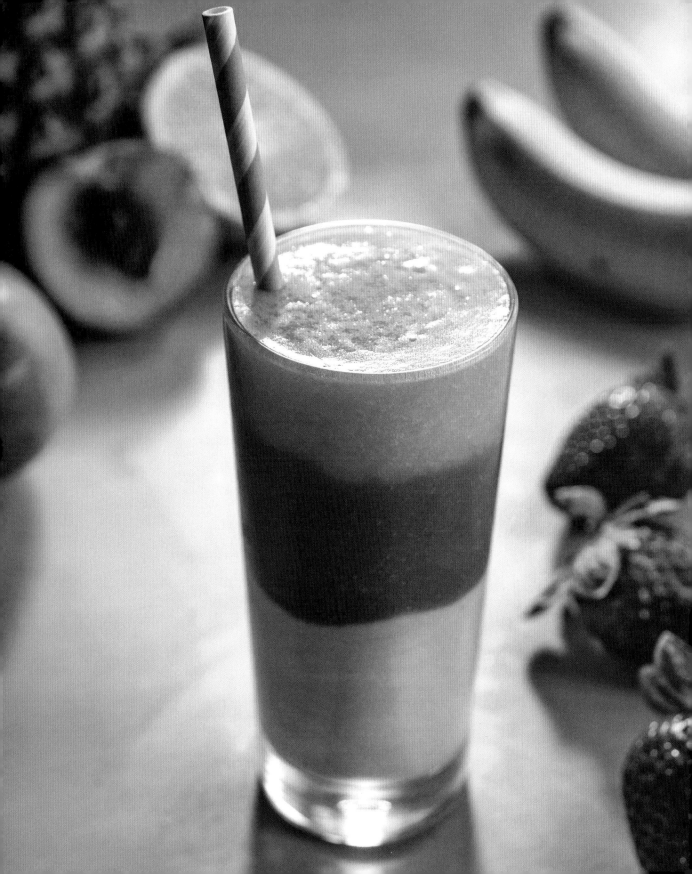

Green with Glow Envy Smoothie

This smoothie will bring out your inner glow, tone and clear up your skin, and make you feel and look amazing. Your friends will envy your new glow. I leave it up to you to decide to share your new beauty secret.

If you like your smoothies sweeter (and trust me, this is already sweet), add an extra ½ cup pineapple.

Makes 2 servings | Serving size: 8 to 10 ounces (depending on how thin you like it)
Per serving: calories 158; fat 5 g; saturated fat 1 g; fiber 6 g; protein 2.5 g;
carbohydrates 28.5 g; sugar 15.5 g | Prep time: 3 minutes | Cook time: 0 minutes

---

1 banana, peeled, sliced, and frozen overnight
1 cup frozen pineapple chunks
½ avocado
1 cup spinach
1 cup chopped romaine lettuce

Place all the ingredients in a blender, add 1 cup water, and pulse. When the mixture starts moving, blend on medium speed until smooth. If you like a thinner drink, add water ¼ cup at a time until you reach the desired consistency. Divide between two glasses and enjoy.

As soon as you've poured the smoothie into your glass, rinse your blender. If you do it right away, nothing will stick and cleaning will be a breeze.

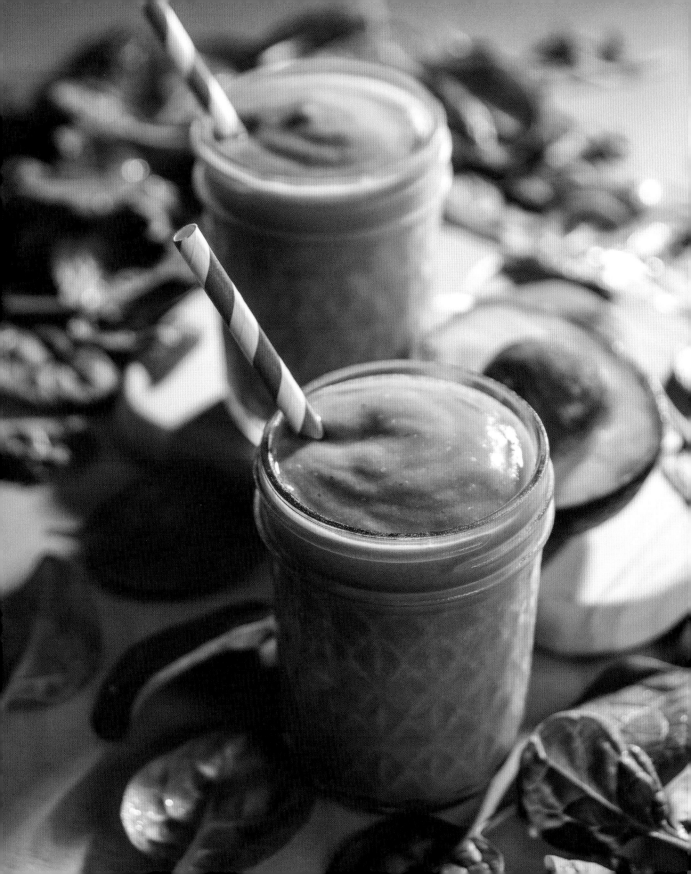

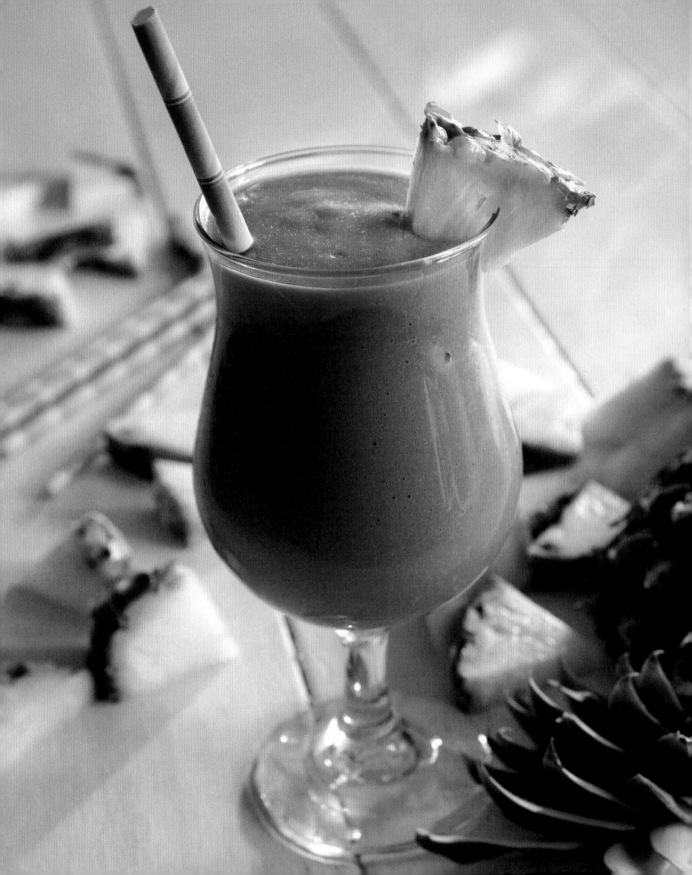

Green Piña Colada Smoothie

Here's a drink that will give you that post-vacation glow! The pineapple and banana both firm up skin, and the coconut oil and greens give you a youthful glow. You'll look and feel beautiful after enjoying this beautifying drink . . . oh, and it tastes like a piña colada, too!

Makes 2 servings | Serving size: 8 to 10 ounces (depending on how thin you like it)
Per serving: calories 136; fat 5 g; saturated fat 4.5; g fiber 4 g; protein 3 g;
carbohydrates 23.5 g; sugar 14 g | Prep time: 1 minute | Cook time: 0 minutes

⅓ cup frozen pineapple chunks
1 banana
1 teaspoon coconut oil
2 cups mixed greens
1 cup unsweetened coconut milk, plus more as
   needed

Place all the ingredients in a blender and pulse. When the mixture starts moving, blend on medium speed until smooth. If you like a thinner drink, add more coconut milk (or water) ¼ cup at a time until you reach the desired consistency. Divide between two glasses and enjoy.

As soon as you've poured the smoothie into your glass, rinse your blender. If you do it right away, nothing will stick and cleaning will be a breeze.

Grown-Up Strawberry Banana Smoothie

One of my most popular blog recipes! Everyone loves a strawberry-banana smoothie, but this one takes the old favorite to a new level with lots of (unobtrusive) spinach. It will taste just like a smoothie you know and love, but that spinach will be boosting your metabolism!

Makes 2 servings | Serving size: 8 to 10 ounces (depending on how thin you like it)
Per serving: calories 179; fat 2 g; saturated fat 0 g; fiber 7 g; protein 3 g; carbohydrates 46 g;
sugar 25 g | Prep time: 1 minute | Cook time: 0 minutes

1 cup frozen strawberries
2 bananas
2 cups spinach
1 cup unsweetened almond milk, plus more as needed
1 teaspoon pure vanilla extract

Place all the ingredients in a blender and pulse. When the mixture starts moving, blend on medium speed until smooth. If you like a thinner drink, add more milk (or water) ¼ cup at a time until you reach the desired consistency. Pour into 2 glasses and enjoy.

As soon as you've poured the smoothie into your glass, rinse your blender. If you do it right away, nothing will stick and cleaning will be a breeze.

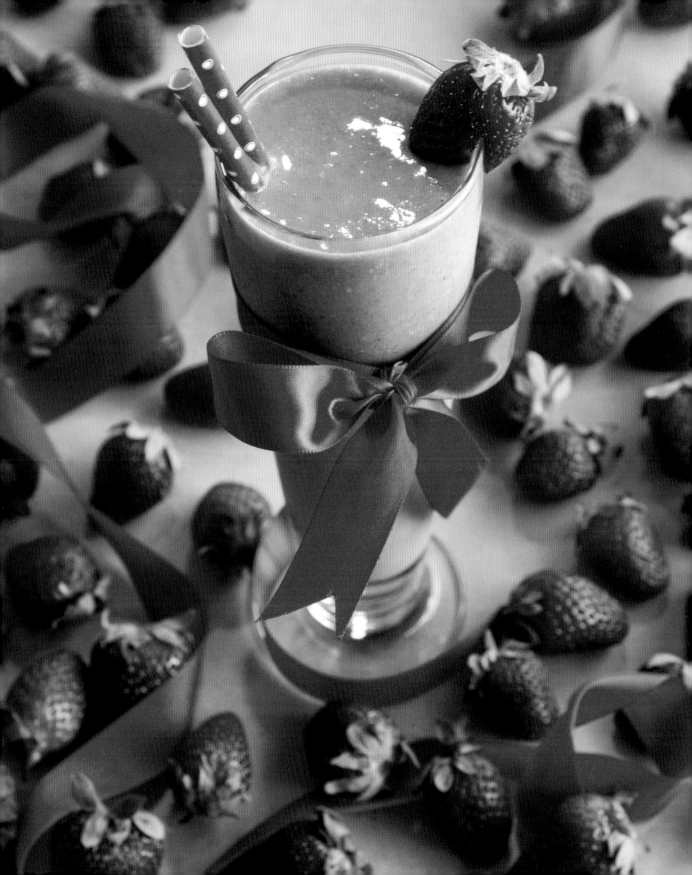

Kale-licious Green Smoothie

As I was wrapping up this cookbook, I realized I didn't have a kale smoothie anywhere in it! And do you want to know why? I don't like kale! I know it's great for me, and I know it's packed full of nutrition, but I find it too acidic and sharp. But I didn't want to get a slew of hate mail for excluding the leafy green, so I started trying recipes and came up with one that I actually love! Yep, I have converted myself into a kale fanatic.

I found that adding milder baby spinach and super-sweet fruits mellowed the harsh raw kale flavor, and I was able to trick myself into eating kale. So the lesson for today is that even foodies and cookbook authors have foods they don't like, but with enough experimentation you can *always* find a way to eat unloved ingredients.

Makes 2 servings | Serving size: 8 to 10 ounces (depending on how thin you like it)
Per serving: calories 89; fat 0.5 g; saturated fat 0 g; fiber 3 g; protein 2.5 g;
carbohydrates 21 g; sugar 15 g | Prep time: 5 minutes | Cook time: 0 minutes

1 cup kale, stems removed
1 cup baby spinach
1 orange, peeled and segmented
½ cup frozen pineapple chunks
½ cup frozen mango chunks

Place all the ingredients in a blender, add 1 cup water, and pulse. When the mixture starts moving, blend on medium speed until smooth. If you like a thinner drink, add more water ¼ cup at a time until you reach the desired consistency. Divide between two glasses and enjoy.

As soon as you've poured the smoothie into your glass, rinse your blender. If you do it right away, nothing will stick and cleaning will be a breeze.

Blueberry Apple Pie Smoothie

This is a super metabolism booster and tastes so delicious that you may feel guilty about drinking it . . . that is, until you look down at its green hue.

My friend Kate is a champion apple pie baker, and years ago she let me in on her sugar-cutting secret—adding blueberries, which lets her get away with using half the sugar. Well, I ran with that, adding blueberries to anything with tart apples—and besides her knock-your-socks-off apple pie, this is my favorite way to enjoy the combo.

Makes 2 servings | *Serving size:* *8 to 10 ounces (depending on how thin you like it)*
Per serving: *calories 84; fat 0 g; saturated fat 0 g; fiber 3.5 g; protein 1 g; carbohydrates 20 g;*
sugar 15 g | *Prep time:* *5 minutes* | *Cook time:* *0 minutes*

1 sweet apple, such as Fuji or Golden Delicious, peeled, cored, and sliced
²/₃ cup frozen blueberries
1 cup baby spinach or mixed greens
¼ teaspoon ground cinnamon
⅛ teaspoon ground nutmeg
1 teaspoon pure vanilla extract
1 tablespoon chia seeds (optional, but this protein addition will thicken it up!)

Place the apple, blueberries, spinach, cinnamon, nutmeg, vanilla, chia seeds (if using), and 1 cup water in a blender and pulse. When the mixture starts moving, blend on medium speed until smooth. If you like a thinner drink, add more water ¼ cup at a time until you reach the desired consistency. Divide between two glasses and enjoy.

As soon as you've poured the smoothie into your glass, rinse your blender. If you do it right away, nothing will stick and cleaning will be a breeze.

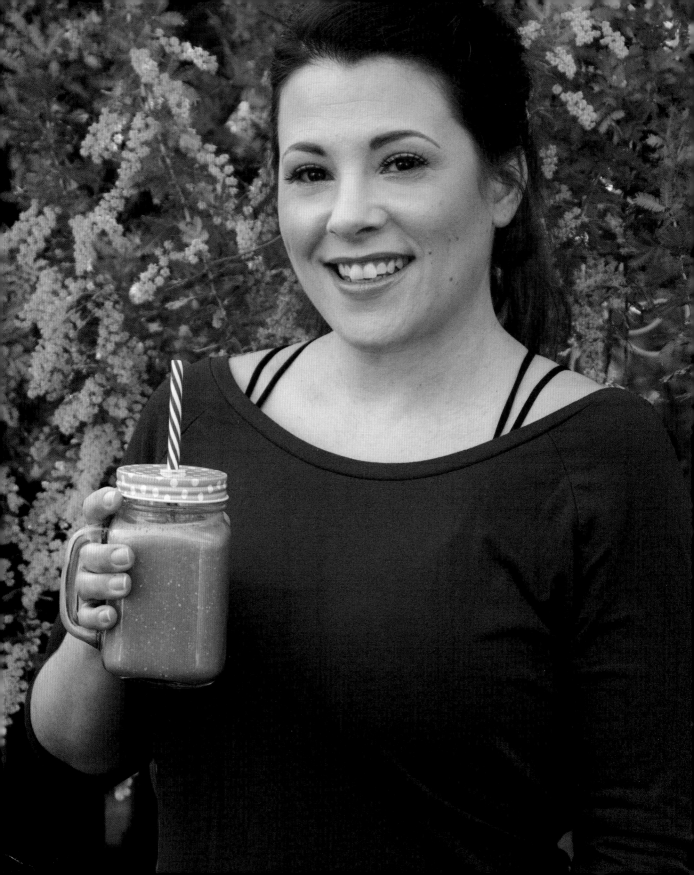

After-Workout Peach Cobbler Smoothie

Packed full of potassium, this after-workout smoothie will help repair muscles for fewer aches and pains after exercise. It also helps firm up muscles and increases collagen health for well-toned body and skin.

Makes 2 servings | Serving size: 8 to 10 ounces (depending on how thin you like it)
Per serving: calories 110; fat 1 g; saturated fat 0 g; fiber 4 g; protein 3 g;
carbohydrates 25 g; sugar 11 g | Prep time: 3 minutes | Cook time: 0 minutes

2 cups baby spinach
½ cup frozen peach slices
1 banana
2 tablespoons old-fashioned rolled oats
¼ teaspoon ground cinnamon

Place all the ingredients in a blender, add 1 cup water, and pulse. When the mixture starts moving, blend on medium speed until smooth. If you like a thinner drink, add more water ¼ cup at a time until you reach the desired consistency. Divide between two glasses and enjoy.

As soon as you've poured the smoothie into your glass, rinse your blender. If you do it right away, nothing will stick and cleaning will be a breeze.

Berry Painless Smoothie

This recipe is perfect for easing aches and pains! Cherries act like "nature's ibuprofen," strawberries relieve nerve pain, and the banana gives a boost of muscle-repairing potassium.

I used two different kinds of greens here, just to get in more nutrients, but if you don't have mixed greens in the house, just use all spinach. Keep it simple, and sticking to the plan will be easier!

Makes 2 servings | Serving size: 8 to 10 ounces (depending on how thin you like it)
Per serving: calories 107; fat 2 g; saturated fat 0 g; fiber 5 g; protein 3 g; carbohydrates 23 g; sugar 12 g | Prep time: 5 minutes | Cook time: 0 minutes

---

5 frozen strawberries
5 frozen cherries
1 small banana
½ cup mixed greens
1½ cups baby spinach
1 tablespoon flaxseeds

Place all the ingredients in a blender, add 1 cup water, and pulse. When the mixture starts moving, blend on medium speed until smooth. If you like a thinner drink, add more water ¼ cup at a time until you reach the desired consistency. Divide between two glasses and enjoy.

As soon as you've poured the smoothie into your glass, rinse your blender. If you do it right away, nothing will stick and cleaning will be a breeze.

Protein-Packed Berry Almond Smoothie

Readers are always asking how they can add protein to green smoothies, and for all these smoothie recipes you can add some Greek yogurt (24 grams of protein per cup). Nuts will add even more protein plus healthy fats. This smoothie has both and is packed with 20 grams of protein!

Makes 2 servings | Serving size: 8 to 10 ounces (depending on how thin you like it)
Per serving: calories 377; fat 11 g; saturated fat 0.5 g; fiber 10 g; protein 20 g;
carbohydrates 57 g; sugar 34 g | Prep time: 5 minutes | Cook time: 0 minutes

1 cup frozen strawberries
1 cup frozen blueberries
2 bananas
2 cups baby spinach
¼ cup unsalted almonds
1 cup 0% Greek yogurt
1 cup unsweetened almond milk, plus more as needed

Place all the ingredients in a blender and pulse. When the mixture starts moving, blend on medium speed until smooth. If you like a thinner drink, add more almond milk (or water) ¼ cup at a time until you reach the desired consistency. Divide between two glasses and enjoy.

As soon as you've poured the smoothie into your glass, rinse your blender. If you do it right away, nothing will stick and cleaning will be a breeze.

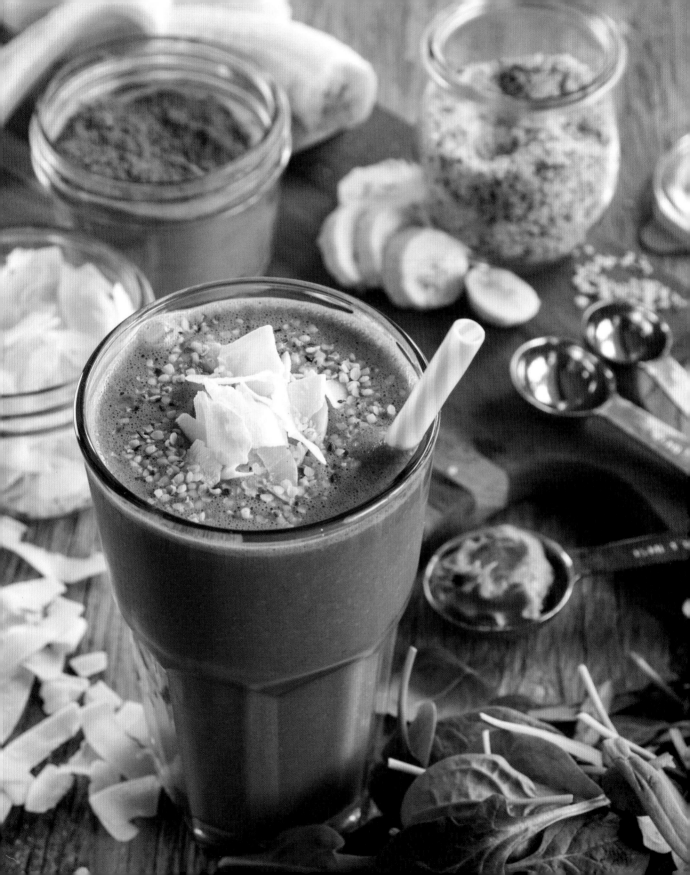

Go Bananas Smoothie

Are you turned off by spotted bananas? Me, too! Next time your bananas start to spot, peel them, chop them, freeze them, and make this smoothie. I like to freeze sliced bananas in individual sandwich bags so that on hectic mornings I can toss the premeasured bananas in the blender with the rest of the ingredients and have a quick and easy breakfast on the go.

Makes 2 servings | Serving size: 10 to 15 ounces (depending on how thin you like it)
Per serving: calories 292; fat 13 g; saturated fat 1.5 g; fiber 8 g; protein 7.5 g;
carbohydrates 44 g; sugar 22.5 g | Prep time: 5 minutes | Cook time: 0 minutes

2 bananas, peeled, sliced, and frozen (do this the night before)

4 cups baby spinach

2 tablespoons almond butter

2 cups unsweetened almond milk, plus more as needed

2 heaping tablespoons unsweetened cocoa powder

1 tablespoon unsweetened coconut flakes (optional)

2 tablespoons hemp seeds (optional)

Place the bananas, spinach, almond butter, almond milk, cocoa powder, and (if using) the coconut flakes and hemp seeds in a blender and pulse. When the mixture starts moving, blend on medium speed until smooth. If you like a thinner drink, add more almond milk (or water) ¼ cup at a time until you reach the desired consistency. Divide between two glasses and enjoy.

As soon as you've poured the smoothie into your glass, rinse your blender. If you do it right away, nothing will stick and cleaning will be a breeze.

Tropical Whirl Smoothie

If you close your eyes, you can almost hear the steel drums and the crashing waves . . . and when you open them you won't even know this is a "green" smoothie! The carrots give this yummy drink a stunning, fancy cocktail–like color.

Makes 2 servings | Serving size: 8 to 10 ounces (depending on how thin you like it)
Per serving: calories 110; fat 2 g; saturated fat 0 g; fiber 5.5 g; protein 3 g;
carbohydrates 22 g; sugar 15 g | Prep time: 1 minute | Cook time: 0 minutes

¼ cup frozen mango chunks
¼ cup frozen pineapple chunks
1 orange, peeled and segmented
2 carrots, shredded
1 tablespoon flaxseeds (optional, but so good for you!)
1 cup coconut water, plus more as needed

Place the mango, pineapple, orange, carrots, flaxseeds (if using), and coconut water in a blender and pulse. When the mixture starts moving, blend on medium speed until smooth. If you like a thinner drink, add more coconut water (or water) ¼ cup at a time until you reach the desired consistency. Divide between two glasses and enjoy.

As soon as you've poured the smoothie into your glass, rinse your blender. If you do it right away, nothing will stick and cleaning will be a breeze.

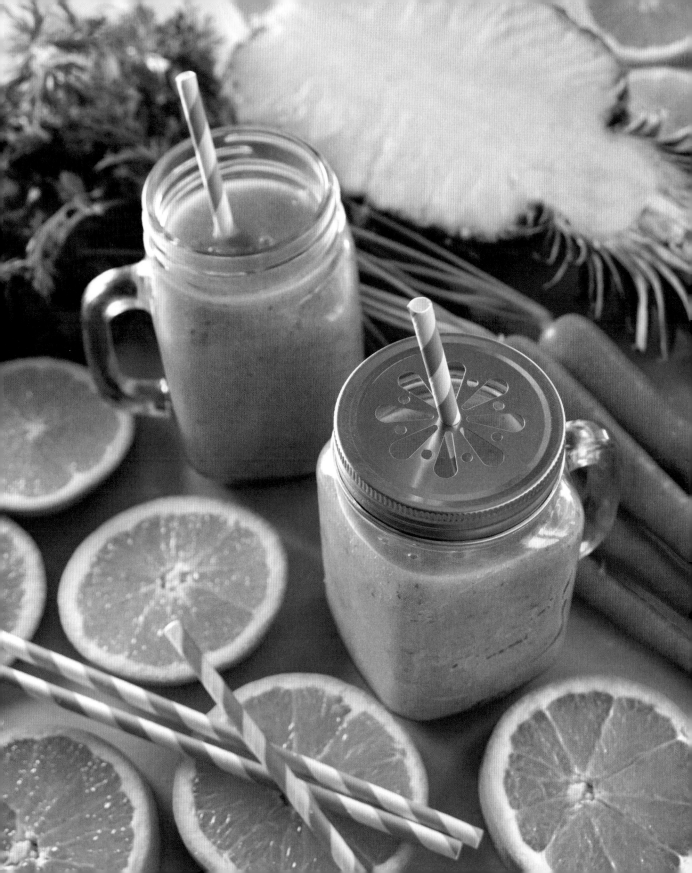

PB&J Green Smoothie

This is one of my go-to smoothies, as I almost always have frozen cherries in my freezer. I love to eat them like frozen grapes, and as a bonus, cherries are a natural pain reliever. So if you suffer from chronic pain (as I do), try out a handful of cherries before you reach for the ibuprofen, or make this smoothie whenever you feel less than fantastic and want to start feeling better fast. For pain management, you want the darkest red cherries you can get.

Makes 2 servings | Serving size: 8 to 10 ounces (depending on how thin you like it)
Per serving: calories 167; fat 5.5 g; saturated fat 0.5 g; fiber 4 g; protein 4 g;
carbohydrates 26 g; sugar 16 g | Prep time: 3 minutes | Cook time: 0 minutes

2 cups baby spinach
½ cup frozen dark red cherries
1 tablespoon all-natural peanut butter
1 banana
1 cup unsweetened almond milk, plus more as needed

Place all the ingredients in a blender and pulse. When the mixture starts moving, blend on medium speed until smooth. If you like a thinner drink, add more almond milk (or water) ¼ cup at a time until you reach the desired consistency. Divide between two glasses and enjoy.

As soon as you've poured the smoothie into your glass, rinse your blender. If you do it right away, nothing will stick and cleaning will be a breeze.

Green "Milk" Shake Smoothie

This creamy smoothie is so velvety and yummy, with avocado, banana, mango, and almond milk adding delicious creaminess. It's the ultimate creamy "milk" shake in green smoothie form!

Makes 2 servings | *Serving size:* 8 to 10 ounces (depending on how thin you like it)
Per serving: calories 171; fat 7 g; saturated fat 0.5 g; fiber 5.5 g; protein 3 g;
carbohydrates 28 g; sugar 18 g | *Prep time:* 3 minutes | *Cook time:* 0 minutes

2 cups baby spinach
½ avocado
½ cup frozen mango chunks
1 banana, peeled, sliced, and frozen (do this the night before)
1 cup unsweetened almond milk, plus more as needed

Place all the ingredients in a blender and pulse. When the mixture starts moving, blend on medium speed until smooth. If you like a thinner drink, add more almond milk (or water) ¼ cup at a time until you reach the desired consistency. Divide between two glasses and enjoy.

As soon as you've poured the smoothie into your glass, rinse your blender. If you do it right away, nothing will stick and cleaning will be a breeze.

3

"Smoothies" for the Non-Smoothie Enthusiast

Hey, friends—I get it. If you've never had a green smoothie before, it might not be that easy to dive in. This chapter is for anybody who's looking to ease into the green-smoothie world. You can use any of these recipes as "smoothies" in the programs in this book, and hopefully they'll help you take the next adventurous step and try some of the green smoothies in chapter 2.

Some of these recipes are very low in calories. If you are using these as a meal replacement, you'll want at least 250 calories, so add a snack from chapter 15, or enjoy two servings instead of one.

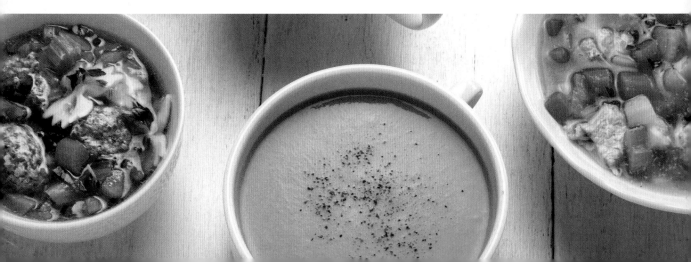

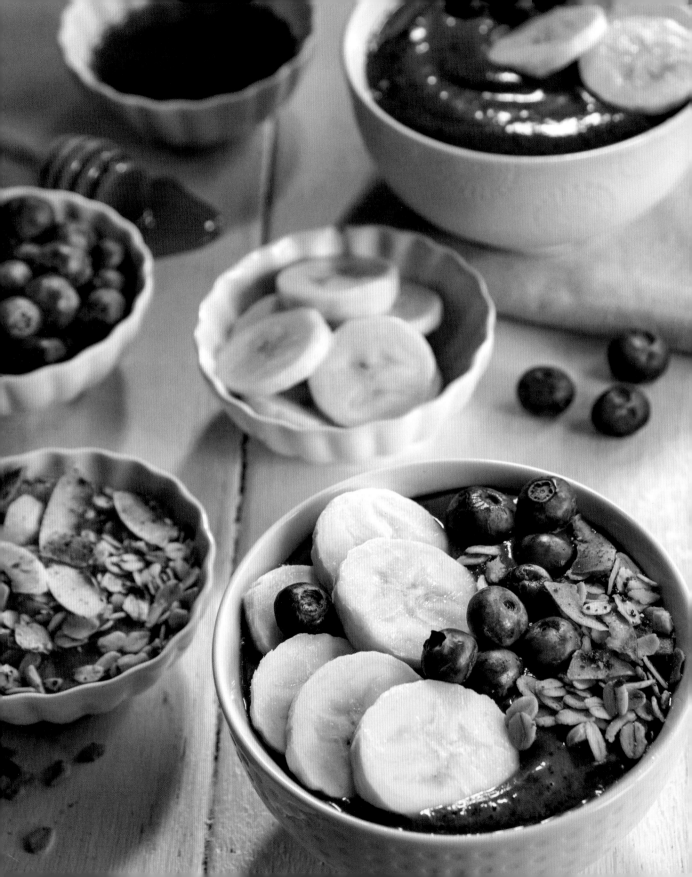

Açaí Bowl with Coconut Granola

I was eating these bright purple bowls before they were fashionable—we're talking ten-plus years ago! I used to get them on my way to work in the mornings, and the smoothie place that made them always put them in tall cups with extra-long spoons. I still like to enjoy them in a cup, so whenever I take these to go, I make them in large lidded mason jars.

I recommend that you make this coconut granola on the weekend or a weeknight so that it will be ready for you in the morning. And if you're gonna make it, you might as well get the ingredients to make the Coconut Banana Parfaits with Coconut Granola (page 214), too, so you'll have two granola-topped breakfasts to alternate for a full week. Saves you time and saves you money!

Makes 2 servings | Serving size: 1 bowl | Per serving: calories 459 g; fat 25 g; saturated fat 3.5 g; fiber 14 g; protein 9 g; carbohydrates 60 g; sugar 23 g | Prep time: 8 minutes | Cook time: 3 minutes

1 orange, peeled and segmented
1½ cups baby spinach
¼ cup unsweetened almond milk
½ avocado
½ cup frozen blueberries
1 (3.5-ounce) packet frozen açaí
½ banana

TOPPINGS
½ banana, sliced
2 tablespoons Coconut Granola (page 214)
2 tablespoons frozen blueberries (optional)
1 teaspoon honey (optional)

1. Put the orange segments in a blender, squeezing them as you drop them in to break them up a little. Add the spinach and almond milk and blend on low speed until smooth. Add the avocado, blueberries, açaí, and banana and blend on low speed until smooth.

2. Divide the mixture between two bowls or mason jars and top with the sliced bananas, granola, and (if using) the blueberries and honey. If you're taking this with you to work, put the granola in a sandwich bag or small travel container and sprinkle it on top when you're ready to eat so it won't get soggy.

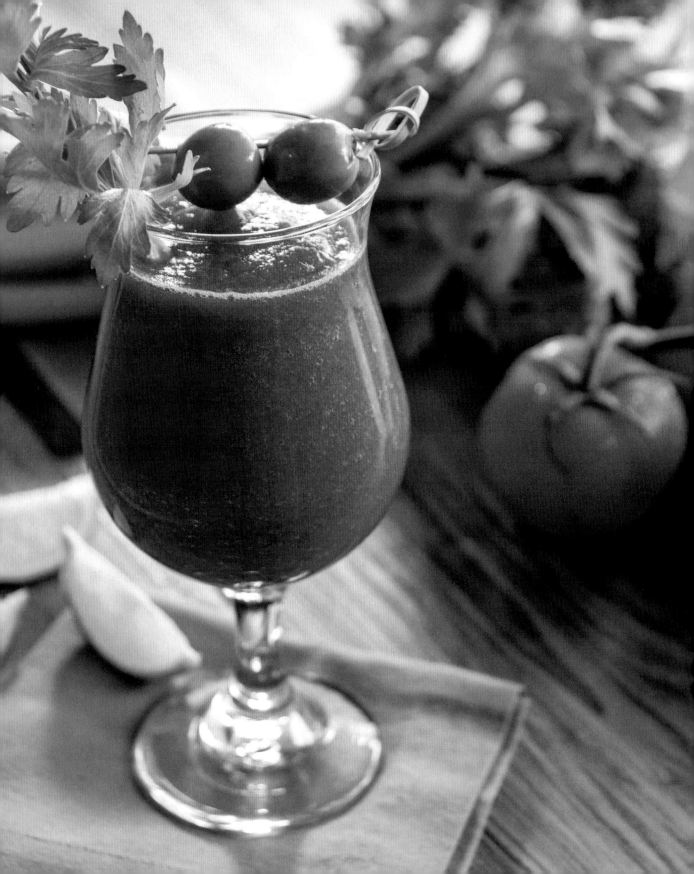

Bloody Mary Mocktail

Here's a great way to take advantage of tomato season! If you're not a fan of the traditional sweet green smoothie, you will love this, and if you're like me and love spicy food, grab your favorite hot sauce now, as it's an optional ingredient!

My all-time-favorite hot sauce is Pepper Plant; I buy it in gallon jugs (and I'm not joking)! It is all natural, contains no preservatives, and works great in any recipe that wants a bit of heat.

But I digress.... Let's get our mocktail on!

Makes 2 servings (or 1 big one if you're feeling extra hungry) | *Serving size: 8 to 10 ounces (depending on how thin you like it)* | *Per serving: calories 50; fat 0.5 g; saturated fat 0 g; fiber 3 g; protein 2 g; carbohydrates 11 g; sugar 7 g* | *Prep time: 5 minutes* | *Cook time: 0 minutes*

---

3 large tomatoes, cored and quartered
4 celery stalks with leaves attached
Dash of Worcestershire sauce
½ cup ice
Pinch of garlic salt or squeeze of fresh lemon juice
Dash of hot sauce (optional)

Place the tomatoes, 2 of the celery stalks, the Worcestershire, ½ cup water, the ice, garlic salt, and hot sauce (if using) in a blender and blend on medium speed until smooth. If you like a thinner drink, add another ½ cup water. Divide between two glasses (or mason jars, for travel) and garnish with the remaining celery stalks.

Piña Colada Ice Pops

Like many of you, I'm sure, I have only one ice pop–mold tray, with just six spots for pops. If that's the case in your house, use wooden ice pop sticks, wrap the frozen pops in wax paper, and move them to a freezer bag; this way you can make all the pops with one tray. They freeze quickly, so it's not too much work!

Makes 9 servings | Serving size: 2 ice pops | Per serving: calories 48; fat 2.5 g; saturated fat 2 g; fiber 0.5 g; protein 2 g; carbohydrates 5.5 g; sugar 4 g | Prep time: 5 minutes plus 2 hours freeze time

2 cups fresh or frozen pineapple chunks
1 cup spinach
½ cup 0% Greek yogurt
1 tablespoon coconut oil
1½ cups unsweetened coconut milk
1 tablespoon unsweetened coconut flakes
(optional)

1. Place the pineapple, spinach, yogurt, coconut oil, coconut milk, and coconut flakes (if using) in a blender and pulse. When the mixture starts moving, blend on medium speed until smooth.

2. Pour into ice pop molds, insert the ice pop sticks, and freeze for 1 to 2 hours, until firm.

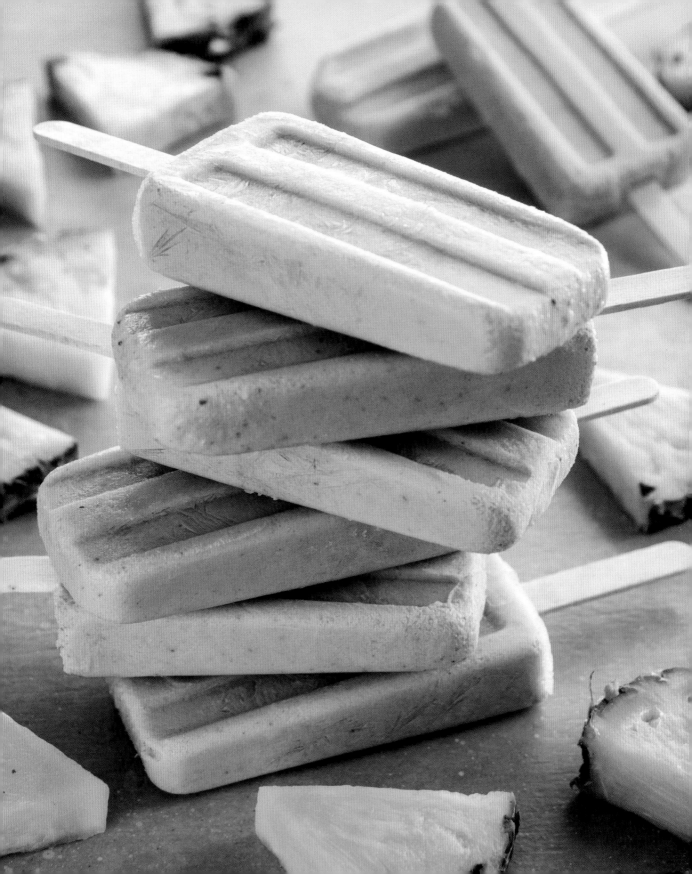

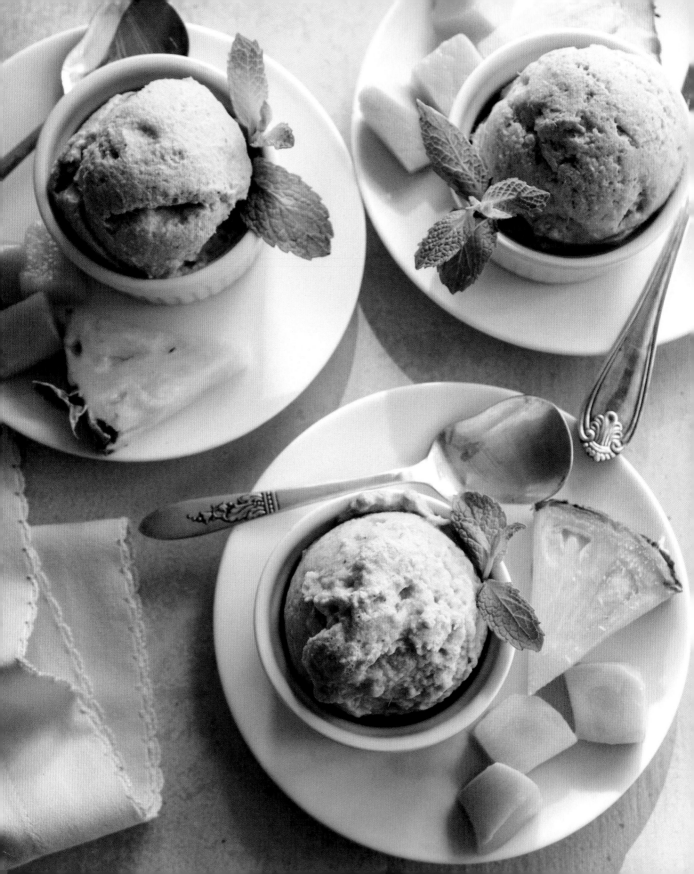

Pineapple Mango Green Sorbet

My daughter went crazy for this sorbet when I first made it. I turned around for a second to get a spoon, turned back, and saw her literally digging her fist into the unfrozen sorbet. She wasn't even an impulse-driven toddler when it happened, but a full-on first grader. Yeah, it's *that* addictive!

Hardest thing about this recipe? Clearing out a spot in your freezer! You must have enough flat space on which to place a filled gallon-size bag.

Makes 4 servings | *Serving size: **about 1 cup** | Per serving: **calories 135; fat 3 g; saturated fat 2.5 g; fiber 3 g; protein 2.5 g; carbohydrates 28 g; sugar 21 g** | Prep time: **15 minutes plus 3 hours freeze time***

1 (10-ounce) bag frozen mango chunks
3 cups frozen pineapple chunks
3 cups baby spinach
2 cups unsweetened coconut milk or almond milk

1. Place the mango, pineapple, spinach, and coconut milk in a blender and pulse. When the mixture starts moving, blend on medium speed until you have a smooth sorbet base.

2. Pour the sorbet into a gallon-size freezer bag and press out as much air as you can without spilling the sorbet all over the counter. Seal and place flat in the freezer for 1 hour.

3. Remove from the freezer and use a rolling pin to very carefully squish and break up the frozen chunks. Repeat this two more times: Freeze for 1 hour, squish. Freeze for 1 hour, squish.

4. Serve the sorbet or transfer it to an airtight container and pack it down well, then cover and freeze for later use. The sorbet will keep for up to 3 months.

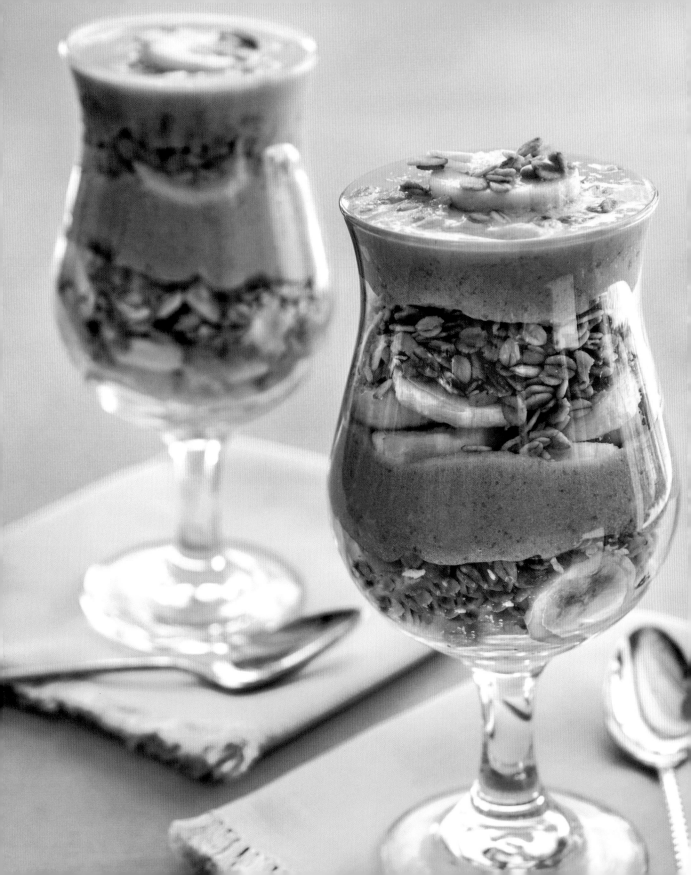

Tropical Green Parfait

Here's another yummy recipe that uses the coconut granola on page 214, so yeah, you gotta get on that and make it soon—it's that good! I tend to use ingredients and base recipes over and over again—it makes things easier and it's important when you're cooking on a budget.

Save yourself time and money and buy frozen fruit; it will keep the consistency thick, and you can enjoy this year-round.

Makes 2 servings | Serving size: 1 parfait | Per serving: calories 304; fat 8 g; saturated fat 3.5 g; fiber 6.5 g; protein 10.5 g; carbohydrates 53 g; sugar 28.5 g | Prep time: 5 minutes | Cook time: 0 minutes

1 cup baby spinach
½ cup unsweetened almond milk
¼ cup frozen mango chunks
½ cup frozen pineapple chunks
1 banana, peeled, sliced, and frozen (but unfrozen will work, too)
½ cup 0% Greek yogurt

TOPPINGS
1 banana, sliced
½ cup Coconut Granola (page 214)

1. Place the spinach and almond milk in a blender and blend on medium speed until incorporated. Add the mango, pineapple, banana, and yogurt and blend on medium speed until smooth.

2. For each serving, add a few banana slices to a glass, sprinkle with 1 tablespoon of the granola, and fill the glass halfway with the green parfait filling. Add more banana slices and granola, then pour on the remaining green parfait filling. Top with the remaining banana slices and granola and serve.

Tomato Basil Soup

Okay, all you green smoothie purists need to bear with me here. Remember, this chapter is for folks who need a little push to drink their veggies. Yes, I know that green smoothies should be raw for maximum benefits, but not everybody's ready for that. If you want a similar recipe in a raw form, check out the Bloody Mary Mocktail on page 49.

This soup is easy and divine, and travels well in a thermos for lunches on the go. Save the leftovers for one of my thirty-minute detox meals, as this soup goes great with the Chicken and Avocado Grilled Cheese sandwiches on page 170.

Makes 4 servings | *Serving size: about 1½ cups* | *Per serving: calories 165; fat 5 g; saturated fat 0.5 g; fiber 8 g; protein 6 g; carbohydrates 29 g; sugar 19 g* | *Prep time: 5 minutes* | *Cook time: 60 minutes*

20 medium tomatoes (I like a combo of Roma and deep red heirlooms such as Beefsteak or Cherokee), cored and quartered
1 large onion, cut into thick rings
4 garlic cloves, halved
1 tablespoon olive oil
3 cups vegetable or bone broth
2 bay leaves
½ cup fresh basil leaves
Freshly ground black pepper
Kosher salt

1. Preheat the oven to 450°F.

2. Place the tomatoes, onion, and garlic in a 9 × 13-inch or larger casserole dish and toss with the oil. Roast for 25 to 30 minutes, until very soft.

3. Transfer the veggies to a large saucepan along with any juices in the baking dish. Add the broth and bay leaves and bring to a boil over medium heat, then lower the heat and simmer for 15 to 20 minutes, until the liquid reduces by about a third.

4. Remove and discard the bay leaves and add the basil leaves. Puree with an immersion blender until smooth. (Alternatively, let the soup cool for 20 minutes and puree in a traditional blender, but be sure to vent the top, as a tomato soup explosion will ruin your day. Reheat in a saucepan before serving.)

5. Simmer the soup for another 10 minutes, then taste for seasoning. Add pepper first, then salt, but only if needed—remember, most broth will be salty enough already. Ladle into bowls and serve hot.

Pesto Pea

Chicken Soup
in a Slow
Cooker

Italian
Wedding

Butternut
Squash

Loaded
Broccoli
Potato

Tomato
Basil

Pesto Pea Soup

As far as I'm concerned, Nigella Lawson knows all, and her words are a cook's gospel. But I have to admit that I changed her recipe a little bit—not because her version isn't excellent (it is) but because it needed more veggies in order to be a good replacement for a green smoothie.

This recipe freezes beautifully. I like to place it in a gallon-size freezer bag and lay it flat to freeze; then when it's frozen solid, it's slim and flat and can fit in even the most packed freezer. To reheat, simply set it out to thaw, add it to a saucepan over medium heat, and cook until hot and bubbling, stirring every 5 minutes.

Makes 6 servings | Serving size: 1 cup | Per serving: calories 124 g; fat 4 g; saturated fat 0 g; fiber 4.5 g; protein 6 g; carbohydrates 16 g; sugar 5 g | Prep time: 5 minutes | Cook time: 10 minutes

3 cups low-sodium vegetable or bone broth
4 cups frozen peas
1 green onion
⅓ cup pesto (see page 107)
½ teaspoon fresh lemon juice

1. In a large saucepan, combine the broth, peas, and green onion and bring to a boil over medium heat. Reduce the heat to a simmer and let it bubble away for 10 minutes. Turn off the heat and remove and discard the green onion.

2. Add the pesto and lemon juice and puree with an immersion blender until smooth. (Alternatively, let the soup cool for 20 minutes and puree in a traditional blender, but be sure to vent the top to prevent a hot soup explosion. Then reheat in the saucepan before serving.)

3. Nigella recommends putting this soup in a thermos for an on-the-go meal, and as usual she is spot on—this soup holds really well throughout the day.

Photo on page 57.

Butternut Squash Soup

I just love butternut squash. The color is stunning, and it's packed with vitamin A, making it a great "beauty food," plus it has lots of potassium for strong bones and muscles.

Sometimes I cut this recipe in half and cube and freeze the remaining squash to use in other recipes, such as the amazing Butternut Squash Wrap on page 108.

Makes 5 servings | *Serving size: 2 cups* | *Per serving: calories 147; fat 1 g; saturated fat 0 g; fiber 3 g; protein 3 g; carbohydrates 35 g; sugar 9 g* | *Prep time: 15 minutes* | *Cook time: 1 hour*

1 (2- to 3-pound) butternut squash, halved and seeded
Olive oil spray
1 medium onion, chopped
3 garlic cloves, roughly chopped
6 cups vegetable or chicken broth
1/8 teaspoon ground nutmeg
Kosher salt and freshly ground black pepper

1. Preheat the oven to 425°F. Line a rimmed baking sheet with foil.

2. Spray the cut sides of the squash with the oil spray and place the squash halves cut side down on the prepared baking sheet. Bake for 45 to 50 minutes, until soft, and set aside to cool.

3. Spray a large saucepan with oil spray and heat it over medium heat. Add the onion and garlic and sauté until the onion is soft and translucent, about 10 minutes.

4. When the squash is cool enough to handle, scoop out the flesh into the saucepan and discard the outer shells. Add the broth, nutmeg, and a pinch each of salt and pepper.

5. Puree with an immersion blender until the soup has a creamy consistency, then crank the heat to medium-high and cook for another 10 minutes. (Alternatively, let the soup cool for 20 minutes and puree in a traditional blender, but be sure to vent the top to prevent a hot soup explosion. Then proceed with reheating in the saucepan before serving.)

6. Taste, add more pepper as needed, and serve.

Photo on page 57.

Chocolate Peanut Butter "Milk" Shake

One of my readers turned me onto PB2, this amazing peanut butter powder that has only 23 calories per tablespoon! It's made by roasting, then pressing the peanuts, which removes 85 percent of the fat and oil. A warning, though: Once you've tasted this stuff, you will become obsessed, especially if you're a peanut butter lover like I am!

Makes 2 servings | *Serving size: about 10 ounces* | *Per serving: calories 295; fat 9 g; saturated fat 1 g; fiber 9 g; protein 16 g; carbohydrates 47 g; sugar 25 g* | *Prep time: 5 minutes* | *Cook time: 0 minutes*

2 bananas, peeled, sliced, and frozen (do this the night before)

4 tablespoons PB2, plus 2 teaspoons for topping (optional)

2 tablespoons unsweetened cocoa powder

2 teaspoons nut butter, such as almond, peanut, or cashew

2 cups spinach

½ cup 0% Greek yogurt

2 cups unsweetened almond milk

Place the bananas, the 4 tablespoons PB2, the cocoa powder, nut butter, spinach, yogurt, and almond milk in a blender and give it a whirl on low speed until smooth. Divide between two glasses and top each with a teaspoon of PB2 (if using). I like to mix it in with a spoon or straw, so when I drink it I get these heavenly little pockets of airy peanut butter.

Cherry Bowl with Chocolate Granola

This bowl is similar to the Açaí Bowl with Coconut Granola on page 214, but with a twist. I wanted to make a bowl for those of you who don't like açaí, can't afford it, or (a common scenario) can't find it at your local stores. I also wanted to create a nerve-healthy meal for all of you who, like me, suffer from nerve pain. This meal will help alleviate most pain, as cherries, especially the dark ones, are known to naturally reduce pain. Oh, and one more difference between the two bowls: This one has chocolate!

This recipe makes more granola than you'll need for two cherry bowls. Just store the leftover granola in an airtight container in the pantry for up to 2 weeks.

Makes 6 servings of granola and 2 servings cherry bowl | Serving size: about 1½ cups cherry bowl and ¼ cup granola | Per serving: calories 359; fat 8 g; saturated fat 3 g; fiber 8 g; protein 18 g; carbohydrates 60 g; sugar 36 g | Prep time: 10 minutes | Cook time: 18 minutes

CHOCOLATE GRANOLA
1 cup old-fashioned rolled oats
1 tablespoon coconut oil
2 tablespoons unsweetened cocoa powder
1 tablespoon semisweet chocolate chips
¼ cup unsweetened applesauce
1 tablespoon raw organic sugar
¼ cup raw sunflower seeds

CHERRY BOWL
2 cups frozen dark sweet cherries
2 cups spinach
½ cup unsweetened almond milk
1 cup 0% Greek yogurt
1 banana, sliced

1. Make the granola: Preheat the oven to 350°F.

2. In a 9 × 9-inch casserole dish, stir together all the granola ingredients with a wooden spoon and spread the mixture evenly in the pan.

3. Bake for 15 to 18 minutes, stirring twice, until golden brown. If you can, leave it uncovered on the countertop overnight to crisp up (but it's fine to serve immediately).

4. Make the cherry bowls: Place the cherries, spinach, almond milk, and yogurt in a blender and blend on low speed until smooth. Divide between two bowls and top with sliced bananas and ¼ cup granola.

4

Easy No-Cook Salads

When it's too hot to cook or you don't have the time or space, this salad chapter is for you—although I think you'll fall in love with these recipes, period! I love that my college-age nieces and nephews can make the salads in their dorm rooms and that when I travel I can quickly throw them together in my hotel room. For other easy meals, check out chapter 8; I created these recipes based on requests I received after my first book came out. Ask nicely and I'll do more fun stuff in book 3!

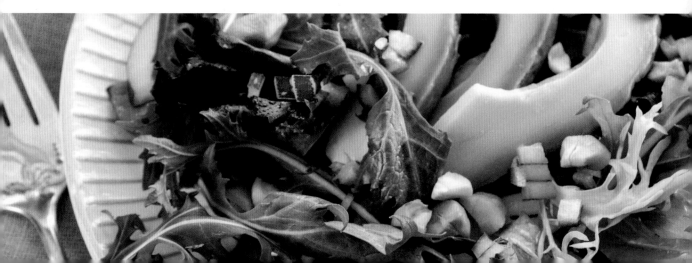

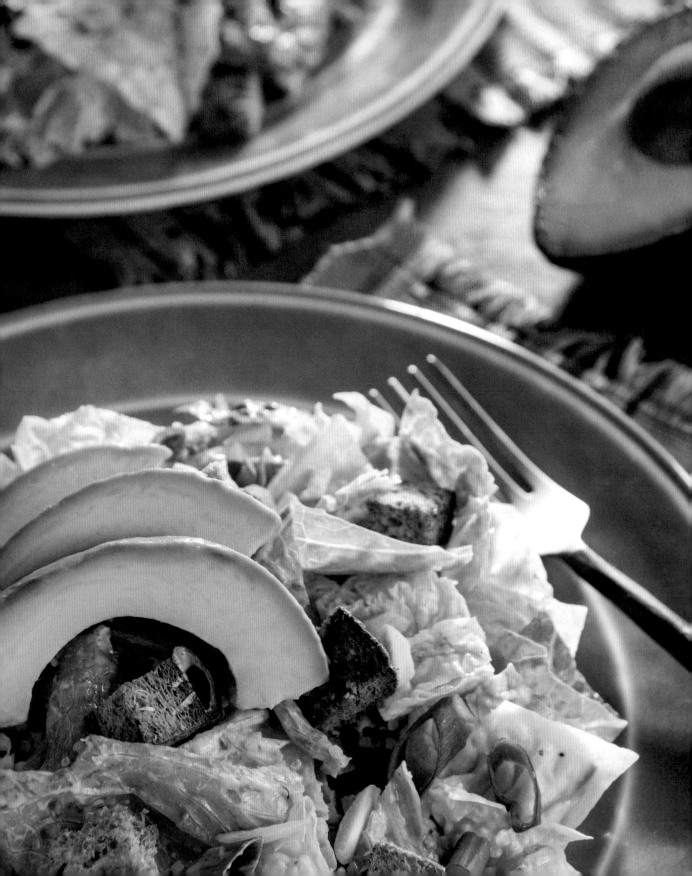

Avocado Caesar Salad

How often do you go out for lunch, hell-bent on getting a fabulous salad, and end up with a mediocre Caesar salad? Sure, once in a while you get a good one, but usually it's so covered in cheese that you're sacrificing health for great taste. Here's what *really* gets me: These run-of-the-mill salads cost $10 to $25, and on average they contain 740 calories!

Here's a Caesar salad that's packed full of flavor, costs less than $5 to make, and has 482 calories, and best of all, there's plenty of cheese flavor! I added the cheese to the dressing so that every single bite contains delicious Parmesan!

Makes 2 servings | Serving size: about 3 cups | Per serving: calories 482; fat 27 g; saturated fat 3 g; fiber 22 g; protein 25 g; carbohydrates 46 g; sugar 18 g | Prep time: 20 minutes | Cook time: 0 minutes

---

2 heads romaine lettuce, chopped

2 green onions, thinly sliced

1 teaspoon slivered almonds

2 teaspoons hemp seeds (optional, but oh so good for you!)

½ cup Caesar Dressing (page 74)

1 avocado, sliced

⅓ cup Homemade Croutons (page 79)

In a large bowl, toss the romaine, green onions, almonds, hemp seeds (if using), and dressing until well coated. Divide the salad between two plates or to-go containers and top with the avocado slices and croutons.

VARIATIONS

- Add some leftover cooked chicken for a chicken Caesar salad.
- Roll up the salad in a large tortilla or wrap for a great salad wrap.

Mediterranean Salad with Sun-Dried Tomatoes

This is my all-time favorite salad—I eat it almost every day for lunch! My family loves it, too, so I often make it as a side dish with dinner. Sometimes I add quinoa, sometimes leftover chicken, and sometimes even avocado. Try it several different ways and find your favorite.

Since this is my go-to lunch, I've mastered the art of making it inexpensive. Here are my tips:

1. Those $5 bins of organic greens you can find at most grocery stores are perfect for keeping salad costs low. They'll save you a ton of money, and the greens seem to last longer than the ones sold in bags.
2. Get a jar of sliced olives—they cost the same as the whole pitted ones and take up less room than whole olives, so you get more for your money.
3. I like the dry bagged sun-dried tomatoes at Trader Joe's. They're cheaper than the soggy jarred ones, have a better consistency, and last longer. I stock up so I don't have to go to two stores in one week—they last forever in your pantry!
4. While you're at TJ's, buy the pine nuts; they're far cheaper there than at a traditional grocery store.
5. Get goat cheese medallions (goat cheese discs). Because they're individually wrapped, you won't end up tossing out soggy goat cheese at the end of the week because air got to your cheese log, again saving you some green.

Makes 2 servings | Serving size: about 3 cups | Per serving: calories 272; fat 19 g; saturated fat 4 g; fiber 3.5 g; protein 8.5 g; carbohydrates 19 g; sugar 11 g | Prep time: 5 minutes | Cook time: 0 minutes

6 cups mixed salad greens
½ cup Greek Mustard Dressing (page 74)
2 tablespoons pine nuts
2 tablespoons chopped sun-dried tomatoes
1 tablespoon sliced Kalamata olives
2 tablespoons crumbled goat cheese

1. In a large bowl, combine the greens, dressing, 1 tablespoon of the pine nuts, 1 tablespoon of the sun-dried tomatoes, and ½ tablespoon of the olives. Toss until the greens are well coated.

2. Divide the salad between two plates and sprinkle the remaining 1 tablespoon pine nuts, 1 tablespoon sun-dried tomatoes, and ½ tablespoon olives on top. Crumble on the cheese and serve.

VARIATIONS

- Make it vegan—replace the cheese with ½ diced avocado.
- Add protein—add cooked chicken or tofu (see page 132 for chicken cooking instructions page 134 for tofu).
- Add fiber *and* protein—add ¼ cup cooked quinoa, then toss with the dressing.

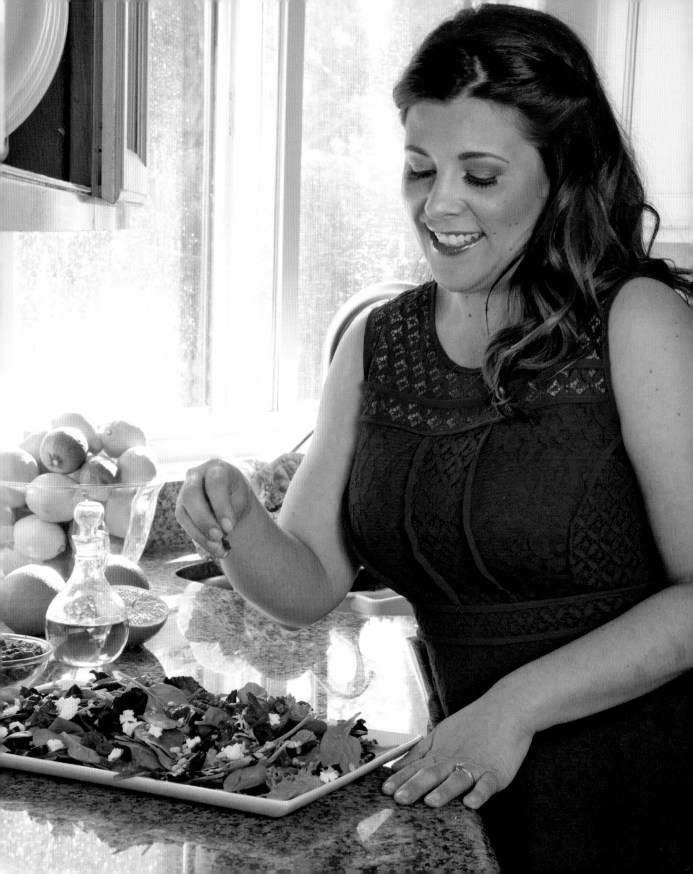

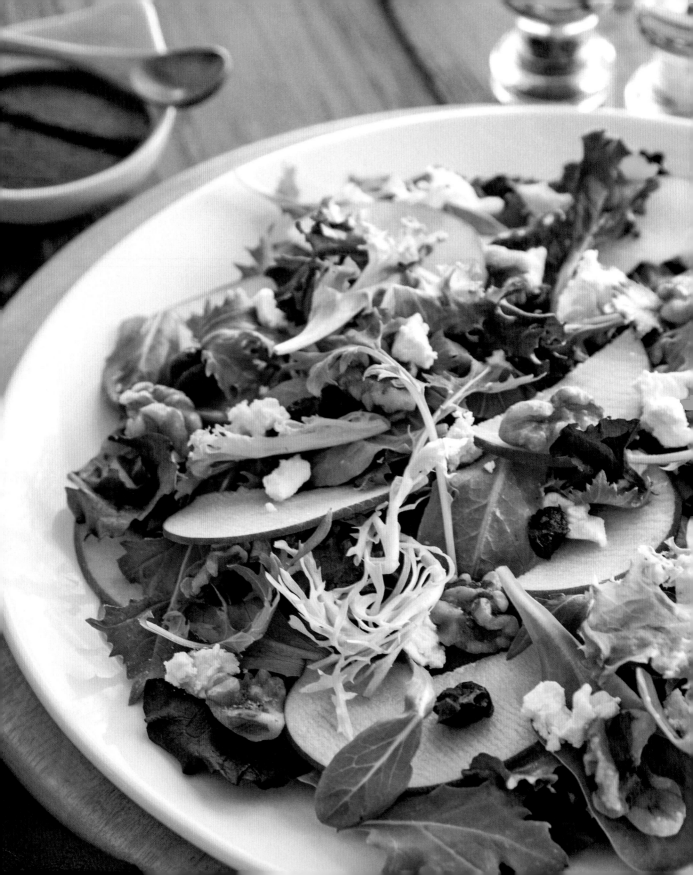

Field Greens with Apples, Walnuts, and Pomegranate Vinaigrette

Here is one of those salads that you end up spending $20 on at a restaurant, and it's usually pretty good . . . but not $20 good! You can make it for about $10 for two salads. It travels well and also makes a great side dish for dinner.

Makes 2 servings | Serving size: about 3 cups | Per serving: calories 305; fat 16 g; saturated fat 3 g; fiber 5 g; protein 5 g; carbohydrates 37 g; sugar 28 g | Prep time: 5 minutes | Cook time: 0 minutes

1 apple, cored and thinly sliced into half-moons
2 teaspoons fresh lemon juice
6 cups mixed field greens
3 tablespoons dried cranberries
2 tablespoons chopped walnuts
¼ cup Pomegranate Vinaigrette (page 76)
1 tablespoon crumbled goat cheese (blue cheese and feta are also great here)

1. In a bowl, combine the apple and lemon juice to keep the apple from turning brown.

2. Divide the greens between two plates or to-go containers for tomorrow and top with the apple, cranberries, and walnuts. Drizzle on the vinaigrette, top with the cheese, and serve.

Summer Salad with Nectarines and Avocado

This easy vegan salad is one of my favorite hot-summer meals. You know those days when it's so hot that chewing makes you sweat, and not only are you avoiding the stove, you're also practically crawling into the fridge? This salad is filling without being heavy and will leave you glowing—in a good way.

If you want to add more protein, some cooked shredded chicken is great on top. See page 132 and make a batch for a week of salads.

Makes 2 servings | Serving size: 3 cups | Per serving: calories 328; fat 24 g; saturated fat 3 g; fiber 7 g; protein 6 g; carbohydrates 27 g; sugar 12.5 g | Prep time: 15 minutes | Cook time: 0 minutes

6 cups mixed greens
1 nectarine, cut into thin crosswise slices
2 tablespoons finely chopped red onion
1 avocado, thinly sliced
¼ cup "Mimosa" Dressing (page 76)
2 tablespoons chopped cashews

Divide the greens between two plates or to-go containers for tomorrow and top with the nectarines, red onion, and avocado. Drizzle the dressing on top and sprinkle with the cashews.

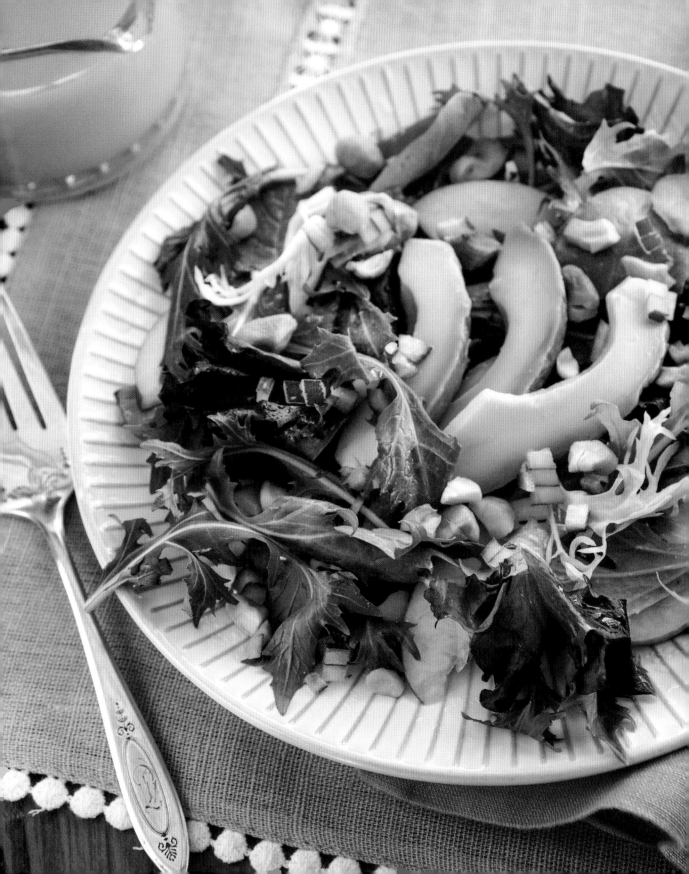

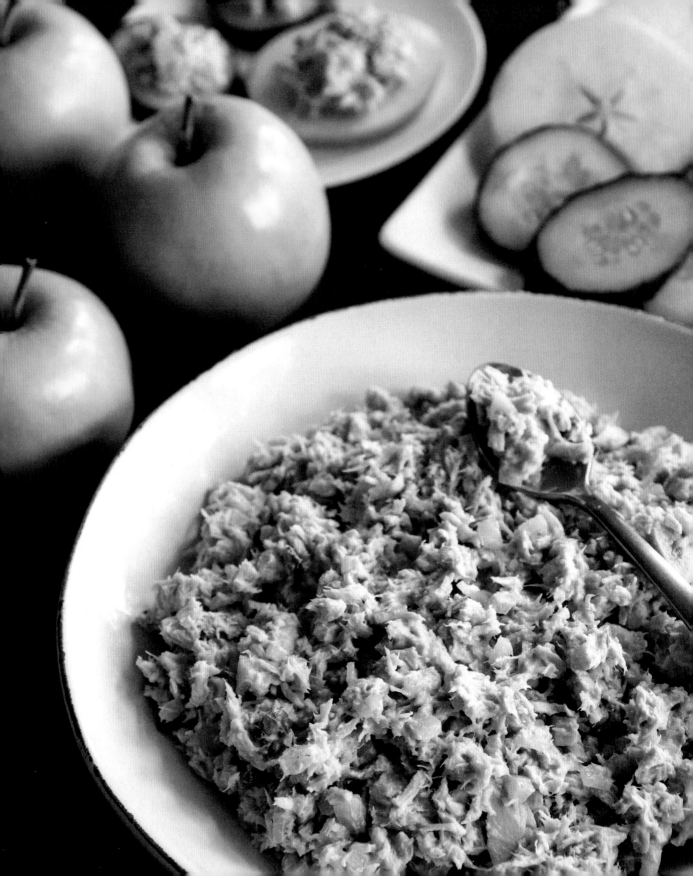

Tuna Salad with Apple and Cucumber Slices

This recipe goes out to my old boss Gina, who made the best tuna salad ever! I used to work in property management (yep, I was a landlord!), and on days that were crazy busy in the office, one of us would run down to our on-site apartment and whip up lunch for the entire staff. Well, Gina always made the best food, and as the boss and the most mature of all us crazy gals, she fed us often!

So what made Gina's tuna salad the best ever? It was the apples! I know that sounds strange, but damn . . . it's so good! But instead of adding the apples to the salad as she did, I use them as tuna delivery devices. I think she'd love my new take on an old favorite.

Makes 2 servings | Serving size: about 1¼ cups tuna salad, 1 apple, and 10 cucumber rings
Per serving: calories 376; fat 6 g; saturated fat 3 g; fiber 5.5 g; protein 48 g; carbohydrates 29 g;
sugar 19 g | Prep time: 8 minutes | Cook time: 0 minutes

1 (12-ounce) can tuna in water, drained
1 green onion, finely chopped
2 celery stalks, finely chopped
¼ cup 0% Greek yogurt
1 teaspoon Dijon or yellow mustard
¼ teaspoon garlic powder
2 tablespoons finely grated sharp cheddar cheese
Kosher salt and freshly ground black pepper
2 green apples, cored and thinly sliced
1 cucumber, sliced into ¼-inch rings

1. In a medium bowl, mix the tuna, green onion, celery, yogurt, mustard, garlic powder, and cheese and season with salt and pepper.

2. Now's the fun part! Spoon the tuna salad on the apple and cucumber slices, or use the slices to scoop the salad. This travels really well and is the opposite of sad desk lunch!

Ten Mason Jar Salad Dressings

These dressings couldn't be simpler or more delicious. For each one, place all the dressing ingredients in a small mason jar, cover, and shake. (Alternatively, whisk together the ingredients in a small bowl and transfer to an airtight container.) Refrigerate for up to 3 days.

The dressings may be used on any of the salads in this book and will also taste great on your favorite homemade salads . . . even restaurant salads! And if you do take one of my salad dressings to a restaurant, please take a photo and send it to me. I will know I have "made it" when someone brings one of my homemade dressing recipes into a restaurant.

Caesar Dressing

This recipe is great with the Avocado Caesar Salad (page 65); it also works well in the Green Goddess Salad Wrap (page 99) if you're looking for an alternative to green goddess dressing.

Make the dressing 1 hour to 1 day ahead of time and refrigerate—the longer it marinates, the better it will taste.

Makes 2 servings | Serving size: ¼ cup | Per serving: calories 67; fat 1 g; saturated fat 0.5 g; fiber 0 g; protein 8 g; carbohydrates 4 g; sugar 3.5 g | Prep time: 2 minutes | Cook time: 0 minutes

2 tablespoons freshly grated Parmesan cheese
1 garlic clove, shredded
½ cup 0% Greek yogurt
2 teaspoons Dijon mustard

1 tablespoon balsamic vinegar
Juice of ½ lemon
Kosher salt and freshly ground black pepper

Greek Mustard Dressing

This is my go-to salad dressing, and I always make it with my go-to salad—the Mediterranean Salad with Sun-Dried Tomatoes (page 66).

You can make this up to 1 day ahead of time, which will intensify the flavor. Before serving, pluck out and discard the garlic clove.

Makes 2 servings | Serving size: about ¼ cup | Per serving: calories 42; fat 2 g; saturated fat 0 g; fiber 0 g; protein 0 g; carbohydrates 4 g; sugar 3.5 g | Prep time: 2 minutes | Cook time: 0 minutes

Juice of 1 orange
1 teaspoon balsamic vinegar
1 teaspoon Dijon mustard

1 teaspoon extra-virgin olive oil (if you have garlic EVOO, use it here—yum!)
1 garlic clove, smashed but still intact

"Mimosa"

Asian-Inspired Peanut Dressing

Easy Homemade Ranch

Avocado Jalapeño

Pomegranate Vinaigrette

Pomegranate Vinaigrette

This vinaigrette makes the Field Greens with Apples, Walnuts, and Pomegranate Vinaigrette on page 69 and the Grilled Steak Salad on page 94 sing. It adds a burst of flavor and would also go well with the Summer Salad with Nectarines and Avocado on page 70, so make extra and enjoy all week long!

Makes 2 servings | Serving size: about 2 tablespoons | Per serving: calories 75; fat 5 g; saturated fat 0.5 g; fiber 0 g; protein 0 g; carbohydrates 7 g; sugar 6 g | Prep time: 1 minute | Cook time: 0 minutes

2 tablespoons balsamic vinegar
1 teaspoon Dijon mustard

¼ cup pomegranate juice
2 teaspoons extra-virgin olive oil

"Mimosa" Dressing

This dressing is the star in my Summer Salad with Nectarines and Avocado (page 70). The citrus perfectly cuts the fat in the avocado and cashews. This dressing may also be paired with the field greens salad on page 69.

Makes 2 servings | Serving size: about 2 tablespoons | Per serving: calories 87; fat 7 g; saturated fat 1 g; fiber 0 g; protein 0 g; carbohydrates 6.5 g; sugar 5.5 g | Prep time: 2 minutes | Cook time: 0 minutes

Juice of ½ orange
1 tablespoon champagne vinegar

1 tablespoon extra-virgin olive oil
½ garlic clove, grated or minced

Creamy "Club" Dressing

This dressing is meant to go with the Club Sandwich Salad on page 83, but you may catch yourself adding it to everything! When we shot the photos for this book, my photographer added it to everything! He drizzled it over the salad it was intended for, a wrap, and some veggies.

Makes 2 servings | Serving size: about 2 tablespoons | Per serving: calories 14; fat 0 g; saturated fat 0 g; fiber 0 g; protein 3 g; carbohydrates 1 g; sugar 1 g | Prep time: 2 minutes | Cook time: 0 minutes

½ garlic clove, grated
¼ cup 0% Greek yogurt
1 tablespoon Dijon or your favorite mustard

¼ teaspoon freshly ground black pepper
2 tablespoons unsweetened almond milk (but any milk will work)

Honey-Mustard Vinaigrette

I just adore honey-mustard dressing, but it's too heavy and can overwhelm a salad. Instead, I opt for a lighter vinaigrette version. Try this on the Fruity Chicken Salad on page 84. Also see page 200 for a creamy honey-mustard alternative.

Makes 2 servings | Serving size: about 2 tablespoons | Per serving: calories 40; fat 2 g; saturated fat 0 g; fiber 0 g; protein 0 g; carbohydrates 5 g; sugar 4 g | Prep time: 2 minutes | Cook time: 0 minutes

Juice of 1 lemon

1 teaspoon extra-virgin olive oil

1 teaspoon balsamic vinegar

1 teaspoon honey

½ teaspoon Dijon or grainy mustard

Asian-Inspired Peanut Dressing

This complex dressing is a great recipe to pull together for a dinner party. Everyone will be extremely impressed that you made something so fancy! It goes with the Chinese Chicken Salad on page 88, which is always a crowd-pleaser.

Makes 2 servings | Serving size: about ¼ cup | Per serving: calories 72; fat 2 g; saturated fat 0.5 g; fiber 0 g; protein 1 g; carbohydrates 5 g; sugar 4 g | Prep time: 2 minutes | Cook time: 0 minutes

1½ teaspoons all-natural peanut butter

1½ teaspoons toasted sesame oil

Juice of 1 orange

1½ teaspoons reduced-sodium soy sauce

¼ teaspoon finely grated peeled fresh ginger, or ⅛ teaspoon ground

Ginger Lime Dressing

I created this recipe to go with the Grilled Veggie Salad on page 92. I had enjoyed a wonderful salad at a local restaurant and wanted to mimic the flavors. That salad had been topped with candied ginger-lime walnuts, but I wanted to avoid those extra calories. So I made this recipe to give that wonderful burst of flavor and kept it simple with raw walnuts, saving time and calories.

Makes 2 servings | Serving size: about 2 tablespoons | Per serving: calories 42; fat 2 g; saturated fat 0 g; fiber 0 g; protein 0 g; carbohydrates 4 g; sugar 4 g | Prep time: 3 minutes | Cook time: 0 minutes

Juice of 1 lime

½ teaspoon finely grated peeled fresh ginger, or ¼ teaspoon ground

1 garlic clove, finely grated

1 teaspoon extra-virgin olive oil

1 teaspoon Dijon mustard

1½ teaspoons balsamic vinegar

1½ teaspoons honey

Avocado Jalapeño Dressing

I promise, it's not spicy!! You remove all the seeds and ribs from the jalapeño, leaving you with a citrus burst and mild heat. I top the Taco Salad on page 95 with this creamy dressing. Think of it like a guacamole dressing—yum!

Makes 2 servings | Serving size: about 2 tablespoons | Per serving: calories 142; fat 11 g; saturated fat 1.5 g; fiber 5 g; protein 4.5 g; carbohydrates 9 g; sugar 2.5 g | Prep time: 5 minutes | Cook time: 0 minutes

1 avocado, smashed
1 garlic clove, grated
¼ cup unsweetened almond milk (but any milk will work)
¼ cup 0% Greek yogurt

1 teaspoon fresh lime juice
¼ cup chopped fresh cilantro
1 jalapeño, ribs and seeds removed, chopped
Kosher salt and freshly ground black pepper

Easy Homemade Ranch

Why fight it—people love ranch! Use this everywhere you love ranch without the guilt, preservatives, sugar, and thickening agents, and feel good about enjoying ranch dressing again! To spice things up, add a tablespoon of salsa to make salsa ranch dressing.

Makes 10 servings | Serving size: ¼ cup | Per serving: calories 30; fat 0 g; saturated fat 0 g; fiber 0 g; protein 5 g; carbohydrates 2.5 g; sugar 2 g | Prep time: 5 minutes | Cook time: 0 minutes

½ garlic clove, minced
3 tablespoons minced fresh chives
2 tablespoons minced fresh flat-leaf parsley
½ teaspoon minced fresh dill
1 teaspoon kosher salt

1 teaspoon freshly ground black pepper
2 cups 0% Greek yogurt
⅔ cup skim milk or unsweetened almond milk
1 tablespoon white vinegar

Homemade Croutons

I always keep the end slices from loaves of bread—they make great croutons! Just place the ends of your bread in a gallon-size freezer bag and toss it in the freezer; add to it and take from it to make croutons as needed. This is a great way to save calories and money, and have you seen how much they are charging for croutons these days? It's just stale bread, people!

Makes 4 servings | Serving size: ¼ cup | Per serving: calories 78; fat 3 g; saturated fat 0.5 g; fiber 1 g; protein 2 g; carbohydrates 11 g; sugar 7.5 g | Prep time: 5 minutes | Cook time: 10 minutes

2 slices whole wheat bread (fresh, frozen, day old; they all work here!)
2 teaspoons olive oil
1 teaspoon garlic salt
2 teaspoons freshly grated Parmesan cheese

1. Preheat the oven to 350°F. Line a rimmed baking sheet with parchment paper.

2. Working over the baking sheet, use kitchen scissors to cut the bread into ½-inch cubes. Drizzle the oil over the bread cubes and sprinkle with the garlic salt and the cheese. Toss to mix and coat and then spread the bread cubes evenly on the baking sheet.

3. Bake for about 10 minutes, until golden brown and crispy. Let the croutons cool on the countertop for 10 minutes; they will crisp up as they sit.

5

Hot and Cold
Meal-Worthy Salads

Boring salads, be gone! Here's a collection of slightly fancy, super-delicious salads–some will even satisfy your craving for a hot meal. All travel well and are yummy at room temperature or cold out of the office fridge, and you'll find that they make great dinners as well.

I love the combination of cool greens and hot veggies or protein—so complex and a great break from the traditional cold salad. Many of these make fantastic side dishes as well—the BYO Beet Salad (page 87), Quinoa and Brussels Sprouts Hot Salad (page 91), and Grilled Veggie Salad (page 92) all make regular appearances on my dinner table alongside a whole roasted chicken (page 190) or crispy pork chops (see page 200).

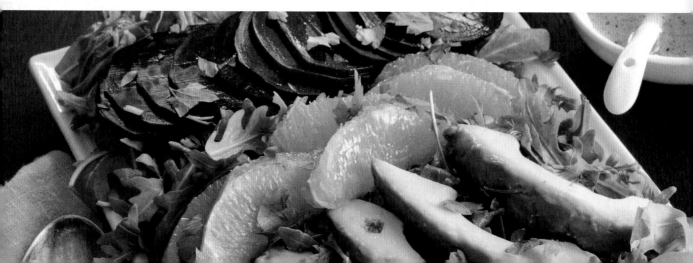

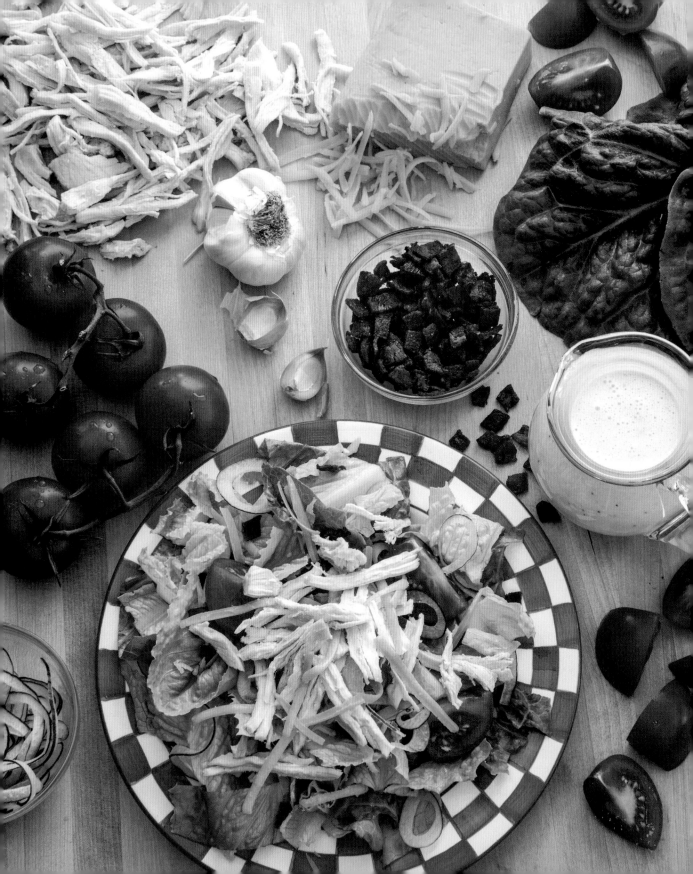

Club Sandwich Salad

Everyone's favorite diner sandwich gets a healthy makeover in this yummy salad!

A note on ingredients: Don't get deli turkey; you want home-cooked, shredded turkey or chicken breast. If you're making this around the holidays, it's a great use for leftover turkey, or check out the directions for cooking a single chicken breast on page 84.

Makes 4 servings | Serving size: about 2 cups | Per serving: calories 285; fat 9.5 g; saturated fat 3 g; fiber 14 g; protein 31.5 g; carbohydrates 27 g; sugar 10 g | Prep time: 20 minutes | Cook time: 8 minutes

4 slices turkey bacon, diced
4 romaine hearts, chopped
1 cup shredded cooked turkey or chicken breast
20 grape tomatoes, halved
¼ red onion, thinly sliced (about 2 tablespoons)
½ cup Creamy "Club" Dressing (page 76)
¼ cup shredded sharp cheddar cheese

1. In a medium sauté pan, cook the turkey bacon over medium heat until browned, about 8 minutes. Transfer to a plate to cool slightly.

2. Divide the romaine among four plates and top with the turkey bacon, turkey breast, tomatoes, and onion. Drizzle the dressing over the salad, then top with the cheese and serve.

Fruity Chicken Salad

I just love salads with fruit in them. Berries add such a great complexity, they naturally increase your metabolism, and best of all, they curb cravings for sweets. If you always have a sweet craving in the afternoon, make this salad for lunch and watch that craving melt away.

When we preempt our cravings with healthy alternatives, we save calories and lose weight. If you don't know what your cravings are, start using the food log on page 21 now. In a few weeks, look back at everything you ate and highlight consistencies. You just may find you crave the same snack every day at the same time. If it's a healthy snack, great, but if you hit the vending machine for something sweet or filled with carbs, feed your body a healthy sweet before the cravings kick in.

Makes 2 servings | Serving size: about 3 cups | Per serving: calories 230; fat 12 g; saturated fat 3 g; fiber 3 g; protein 17.5 g; carbohydrates 14 g; sugar 8 g | Prep time: 15 minutes | Cook time: 10 minutes

CHICKEN
1 boneless, skinless chicken breast
1 teaspoon olive oil
¼ teaspoon garlic salt
¼ teaspoon freshly ground black pepper

SALAD
6 cups baby spinach
¼ cup fresh blueberries
½ cup hulled and sliced fresh strawberries
1 tablespoon chopped walnuts
¼ cup Honey-Mustard Vinaigrette (page 77)
1 tablespoon crumbled goat cheese

1. Make the chicken: Brush the chicken with the oil and sprinkle it with the garlic salt and pepper. Heat a small skillet over medium-high heat and add the chicken. Cook, covered, for 4 to 6 minutes per side, until cooked through (no pink on the inside and the juices run clear). Transfer to a plate to cool, then cut it into ¼-inch dice.

2. Make the salad: In a large bowl, combine the spinach, blueberries, strawberries, walnuts, dressing, and half the chicken. Add the dressing and toss well to coat.

3. Transfer the salad to two plates or to-go containers for tomorrow and top evenly with the remaining chicken and the goat cheese.

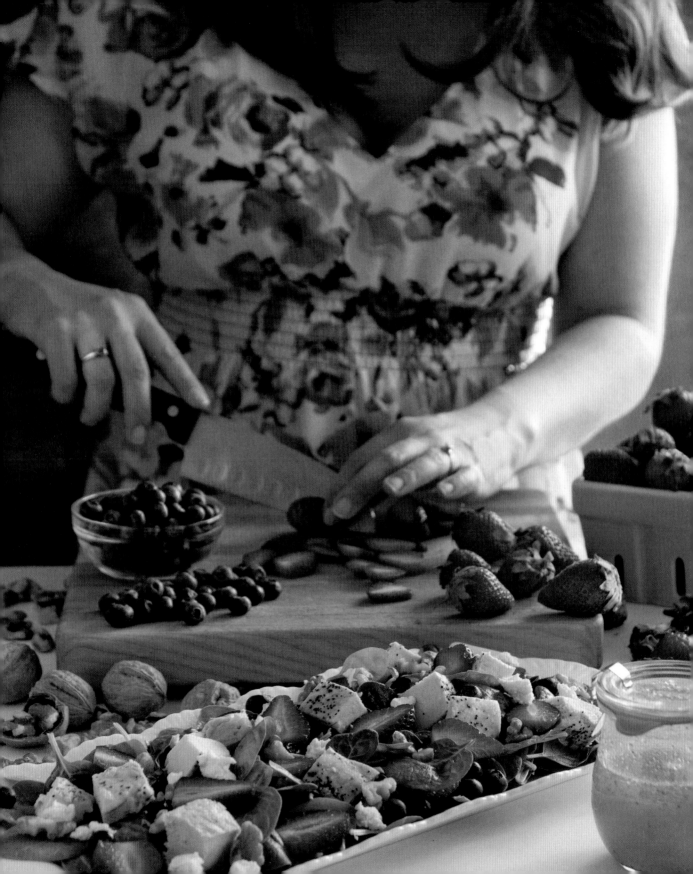

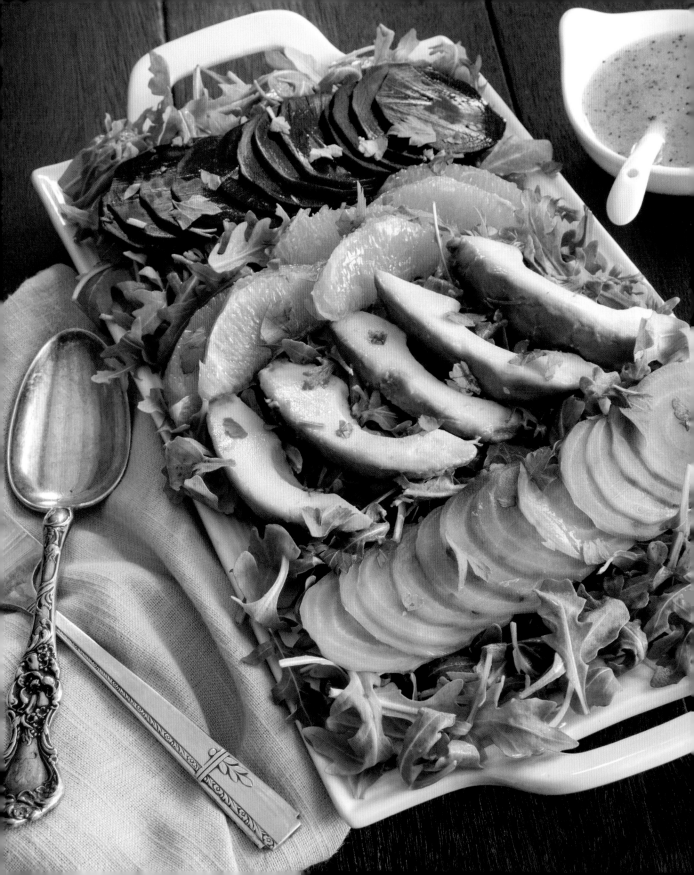

BYO Beet Salad

I really love this salad, which is modified slightly from a yummy beet salad on my blog. Beets have a very earthy flavor, and some people complain that they taste like dirt, but if you make them right, they're divine—and they're so good for you!

I use lots of citrus to help cut the earthy flavor, and with the creaminess of the avocados this salad will turn any beet hater into a beet lover.

Makes 2 servings | Serving size: about 2 cups | Per serving: calories 429; fat 25 g; saturated fat 3 g; fiber 15 g; protein 6 g; carbohydrates 53 g; sugar 37 g | Prep time: 30 minutes | Cook time: 60 minutes

3 large beets
2 tablespoons olive oil
Kosher salt and freshly ground black pepper
2 cups arugula
2 oranges, peeled and segmented
¼ cup "Mimosa" Dressing (page 76)
1 avocado, sliced
⅓ cup fresh flat-leaf parsley leaves

1. Preheat the oven to 450°F. Line a 9 × 9-inch casserole dish with 2 feet of foil.

2. Cut the ends off the beets and scrub them clean. Place the beets in the prepared casserole dish. Cover with the oil and season with salt and pepper. Close up the foil and seal the ends, leaving room for air inside the foil packet. Roast for 1 hour, or until the beets are soft when you pierce them with a fork. Remove the beets from the oven and let cool, then open the packet and move the beets to a cutting board (use plastic—beets will stain wood).

3. When the beets are cool enough to handle, use a paper towel to help remove the skins—just wipe them off. Cut the beets into very thin slices.

4. Divide the arugula between two plates. Top with the beets, then the orange segments. Pour the dressing over the salads, then top with the avocado. Use a pair of scissors to snip the parsley over the plates. Serve hot or cold.

Chinese Chicken Salad

Gone are the days of boring old Chinese chicken salads with fried toppings. Honestly, friends, they're not that healthy or even great-tasting! But this one is extremely healthy and filling, and don't fret over the lack of fried wontons or noodles—it's plenty crunchy!

You can easily make this a vegan dish by omitting the chicken; add 1 to 2 tablespoons of chopped peanuts for extra protein and a healthy dose of good fats.

Makes 2 servings | Serving size: 3 cups | Per serving: calories 394; fat 16 g; saturated fat 2 g; fiber 10 g; protein 25 g; carbohydrates 36 g; sugar 8 g | Prep time: 15 minutes | Cook time: 15 minutes

¼ cup uncooked quinoa
Olive oil spray
1 boneless, skinless chicken breast
Kosher salt and freshly ground black pepper
3 cups chopped romaine lettuce
2 large carrots, shredded
2 cups shaved Brussels sprouts
2 green onions, thinly sliced
1 tablespoon slivered almonds
1 tablespoon sesame seeds
1 tablespoon hemp seeds (optional)
½ cup Asian-Inspired Peanut Dressing
    (page 77)

1. Rinse the quinoa with cold water (to take out the bitterness), then place in a small saucepan over medium heat. Cover with ½ cup water and simmer, covered, until all the water is absorbed, about 10 minutes.

2. Lightly spray a medium skillet with oil spray and place over medium heat. Sprinkle the chicken breast with a pinch each of salt and pepper and cook, covered, for 4 to 6 minutes on each side, until cooked through and the juices run clear.

3. In a large bowl, combine the romaine, carrots, Brussels sprouts, green onions, almonds, sesame seeds, hemp seeds (if using), and the cooked quinoa.

4. Cut the chicken into bite-size cubes and add it to the salad.

5. Drizzle the dressing over the salad, toss it all together, and serve.

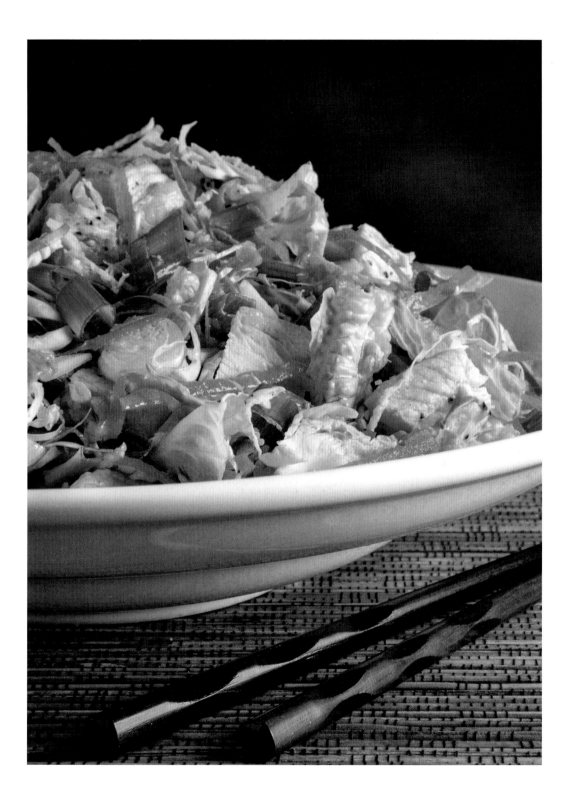

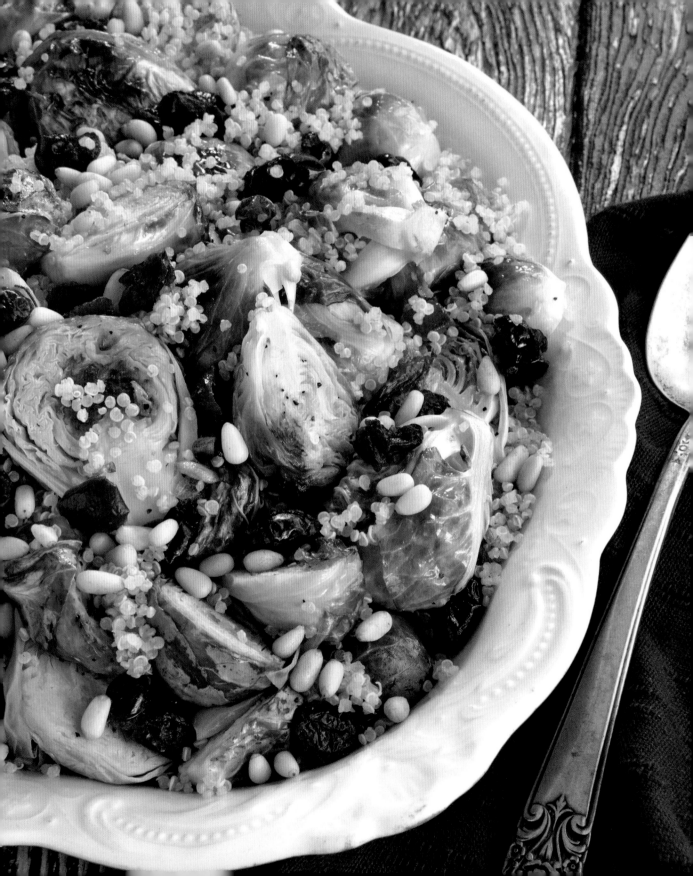

Quinoa and Brussels Sprouts Hot Salad

Yum, I love this recipe! It's inspired by a wonderful vegan blog called *Thug Kitchen*. I made it a few years back as a holiday side dish and have been playing with the recipe ever since. I've changed it up quite a bit, but I simply must give credit where credit is due . . . so, thanks, *Thug Kitchen*—you rock!

P.S. This makes a great side dish or full meal and goes really well with a turkey or chicken dinner!

Makes 2 servings | Serving size: about 2 cups | Per serving: calories 370; fat 16 g; saturated fat 1 g; fiber 11.5 g; protein 13 g; carbohydrates 50.5 g; sugar 17 g | Prep time: 20 minutes | Cook time: 30 minutes

---

1 pound Brussels sprouts, dark outer leaves removed, halved lengthwise
2 tablespoons minced yellow onion
1 garlic clove, chopped
1 teaspoon olive oil
¼ cup uncooked quinoa
2 tablespoons chopped dried cranberries
2 tablespoons pine nuts
¼ cup Honey-Mustard Vinaigrette (page 77)

1. Preheat the oven to 350°F.

2. In a 9 × 13-inch casserole dish, toss together the Brussels sprouts, onion, garlic, and oil. Bake for 30 minutes, or until lightly browned and tender, stirring once to avoid burning.

3. Meanwhile, rinse the quinoa with cold water (to take out the bitterness), then place in a small saucepan. Cover with ½ cup water and simmer, covered, over medium heat until all the water is absorbed, about 10 minutes.

4. In a large bowl, combine the Brussels sprouts mixture, quinoa, cranberries, pine nuts, and dressing. Toss together and serve.

Grilled Veggie Salad

There is this tiny beer bar in my town that makes hands down the best vegetarian food I've ever had! I know, sounds strange, right? But I figure if I'm gonna have a beer I might as well eat healthy. At first I found ordering a vegetarian meal to be a downer—I was celebrating and I wanted something over-the-top naughty—but I was good and got a grilled veggie salad, and now I crave it weekly! It's saying a lot when I pass up their bacon mac and cheese, bangers and mash, and homemade Bavarian pretzels for a *salad*!

So of course I had to re-create it and share it here. I recommend you enjoy it with some sparkling water—so yummy with the bubbles and, unlike beer, no calories.

Makes 2 servings | Serving size: about 3 cups | Per serving: calories 227; fat 12 g; saturated fat 3 g; fiber 4 g; protein 7 g; carbohydrates 19 g; sugar 5 g | Prep time: 20 minutes | Cook time: 20 minutes

1 medium zucchini, thinly sliced into 2-inch sticks
½ red onion, thinly sliced
1 red bell pepper, cut into thin strips
1 cup sliced white mushrooms
1 garlic clove, smashed but still intact
1 teaspoon olive oil
Kosher salt and freshly ground black pepper
4 cups mixed salad greens
¼ cup Ginger Lime Dressing (page 77)
2 tablespoons crumbled reduced-fat feta cheese
2 tablespoons roughly chopped walnuts

1. In a large grill pan or sauté pan, toss together the zucchini, onion, bell pepper, mushrooms, garlic clove, oil, and a pinch each of salt and pepper and cook over medium heat for 15 to 20 minutes, stirring often, until the vegetables are soft. Remove and discard the garlic.

2. To serve, top two plates with the greens and divide the cooked vegetables between the plates. Drizzle the dressing on top, then sprinkle on the feta and walnuts and serve.

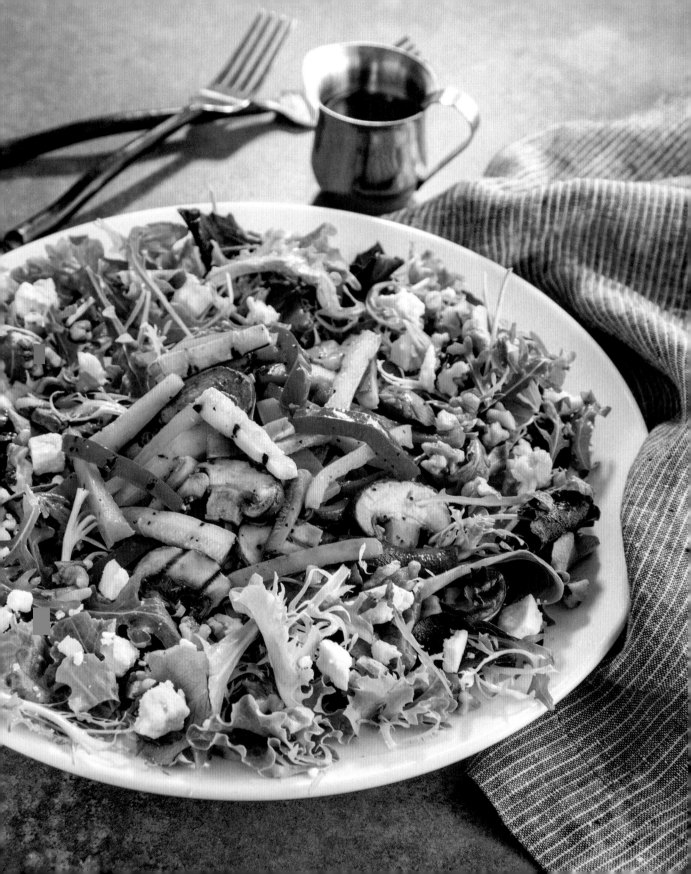

Grilled Steak Salad

Getting your family to eat a salad can be difficult, but a steak salad is harder to turn down, so next time you want to get them to eat their greens, tempt them with this. You can use leftover steak here—it's a great way to save money.

Makes 2 servings | *Serving size: about 2 cups* | *Per serving: calories 369; fat 20 g; saturated fat 6 g; fiber 4 g; protein 28 g; carbohydrates 20 g; sugar 9 g* | *Prep time: 20 minutes* | *Cook time: 25 minutes*

⅛ teaspoon sea salt
⅛ teaspoon freshly ground black pepper
¼ teaspoon cayenne
2 teaspoons garlic powder
1 (1-pound) sirloin steak, about 1 inch thick
Olive oil spray
4 asparagus spears, ends trimmed
4 cups baby spinach
2 cups arugula
1 tomato, cut into bite-size pieces
1 cup frozen corn, thawed
½ cup Pomegranate Vinaigrette (page 76)
¼ cup crumbled goat cheese
¼ cup fresh basil leaves, torn

1. Preheat the oven to 350°F.

2. In a small bowl, combine the salt, pepper, cayenne, and garlic powder and mix well. Rub the mixture on both sides of the steak, cover the steak in plastic wrap, and refrigerate for 1 hour or up to overnight.

3. Spray a ridged cast-iron pan (or other oven-safe pan) with oil spray and place over medium-high heat. Grill the steak for 5 to 6 minutes on each side, until browned. Place the pan in the oven and let the steak cook for 10 to 15 minutes, less if it is a thinner cut, until browned and red in the center. When the steak is done, let it rest for 10 minutes to keep it tender and juicy.

4. Using a vegetable peeler, peel the asparagus into long strips.

5. Rip up the spinach leaves and place them in a large bowl. Top with the arugula, asparagus strips, tomato, and corn. Drizzle the dressing over the salad. Thinly slice the steak and arrange on top. Sprinkle the cheese over the salad, garnish with some torn basil, and serve.

Taco Salad

Halfway through writing this book, we moved from California to Boise, Idaho. Now, I don't want to say the Mexican food in Idaho is bad (I probably just haven't found the right place yet), but I can say that it doesn't hold a candle to Cali's abundance of amazing Mexican food.

I ordered a taco salad at a local restaurant here and it was served in a deep-fried shell that was dripping with oil, had hardly any vegetables, and was covered in cheese sauce. It was neither healthy nor tasty, and I couldn't even stomach it. I went home with a mean craving for a healthy, light taco salad, so I went to my kitchen and this yummy recipe was born.

Makes 2 servings | Serving size: 1 bowl | Per serving: calories 468; fat 28 g; saturated fat 9.5 g; fiber 30 g; protein 30 g; carbohydrates 42 g; sugar 5 g | Prep time: 20 minutes | Cook time: 30 minutes

2 (8-inch) whole wheat tortillas
Olive oil spray
1 small onion, finely chopped
Pinch of kosher salt
¼ pound ground turkey
1½ teaspoons chili powder
½ teaspoon cayenne
1½ teaspoons garlic powder
½ teaspoon dried oregano
3 cups chopped romaine lettuce
1 tomato, cut into medium dice
1 green onion, thinly sliced
¼ cup frozen corn, thawed
¼ cup Avocado Jalapeño Dressing (page 78)
2 tablespoons sliced canned black olives
2 tablespoons shredded sharp cheddar cheese

1. Preheat the oven to 375°F.

2. Place the tortillas in two oven-safe bowls (or use two 9 × 9-inch casserole dishes and ball up some foil in the corners of the dish to give it a bit of a bowl shape). Spray the tops of the tortillas lightly with oil and bake for 10 to 20 minutes, until you have browned, crispy tortilla bowls.

3. Meanwhile, spray a sauté pan with oil spray and place it over medium heat. Add the onion and salt and sauté for 10 minutes, or until the onion is soft. Add the turkey and cook for 10 minutes, or until browned, breaking it up as it cooks.

4. Add the chili powder, cayenne, garlic powder, oregano, and ¼ cup water. Mix well and cook for about 10 minutes more, until the turkey is cooked and most of the liquid is absorbed.

5. Transfer the tortilla bowls to two plates and fill them with the romaine, tomato, green onion, corn, and turkey. Drizzle the dressing on top and sprinkle evenly with the olives and cheese.

6

That's a Wrap . . . Salad Wraps!

Long ago I discovered that salad wrapped in a large tortilla was a delicious way to enjoy leftovers, especially the next day when the dressing has made the salad a little soggy. It's a great way to salvage your leftovers and save money.

This chapter gives you salads that make you feel like you're getting much more than just a plate of greens. They're all perfect for your detox salad meals, so dig in when you're bored with salads or just want to try something new. My favorite is the Spring Rolls with Peanut Sauce; I make them weekly and have to hide half of them in the back of the fridge so I don't eat them all in one sitting.

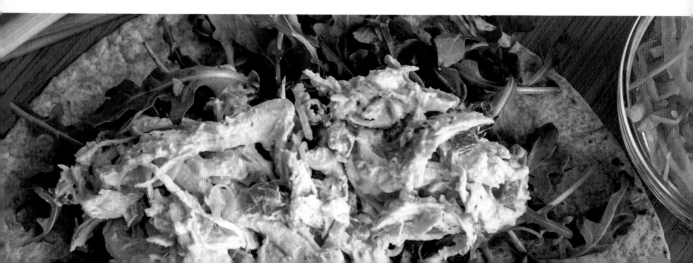

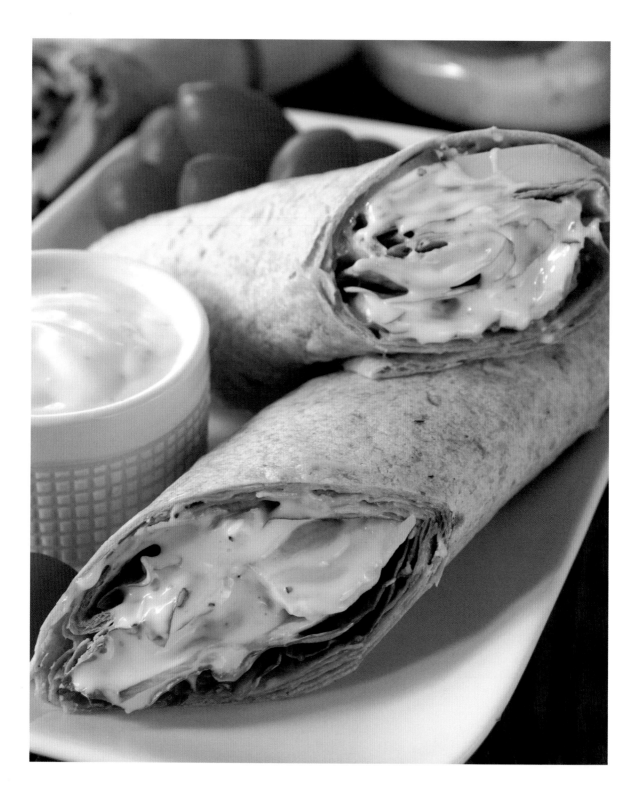

Green Goddess Salad Wrap

Okay, if you're a longtime reader of my blog, you may want to sit down—I broke one of my own rules here! For years now, I have begged people to stop buying store-bought salad dressing. I still believe it's a huge waste of money, and most of them are packed full of preservatives and chemicals that will hinder your weight-loss efforts. But I figured with so many salads and salad wraps in this book, I might as well throw you all a bone and share a good alternative for making your own (which I still really recommend you do). Annie's organic green goddess dressing is not only one of the most popular on the market but also okay to enjoy on all the salads on my program.

When you're prepping this recipe, go ahead and slice up the whole bell pepper and cucumber and throw them in the fridge, ready for tomorrow!

Makes 1 serving | Serving size: 1 wrap | Per serving: calories 398; fat 21 g; saturated fat 4 g; fiber 9 g; protein 8 g; carbohydrates 47 g; sugar 5 g | Prep time: 5 minutes | Cook time: 0 minutes

---

1 (10-inch) burrito-size spinach wrap (looks like a green tortilla; you'll find it by the tortillas or bread)

2 romaine leaves

½ avocado, thinly sliced

¼ bell pepper, sliced into thin strips (I like green here, but any color will work)

1 (1-inch) piece cucumber, sliced into thin rings

1 tablespoon Annie's organic green goddess dressing or Easy Homemade Ranch (page 78)

1. Place the spinach wrap on a clean surface (or on parchment paper, if you're wrapping it to go) and top with the romaine leaves, avocado, bell pepper, and cucumber. Add the dressing if you're eating it now, or put it in a container to add later so the wrap stays fresh.

2. Wrap up the spinach wrap like you're folding a letter—fold one-third over the middle third and the remaining third over that, overlapping in the center—cut in half, and dig in.

Spring Rolls with Peanut Sauce

I was so nervous to work with rice paper until I finally tried it out. Boy, do I feel silly for waiting so long! After making two spring rolls, my seven-year-old took over. No, I'm not kidding—she's fearless and kicked me out of my own kitchen. If a first-grader can do it, so can you. Just dive in!

One tip: If the rice paper starts sticking together (like tape does at the worst possible moment), just drop it back in the water—it will unstick in seconds and you can start over! Now, if only that worked with tape....

Makes 2 servings | *Serving size: 4 spring rolls* | *Per serving: calories 361; fat 16 g; saturated fat 2.5 g; fiber 3.5 g; protein 9.5 g; carbohydrates 40.5 g; sugar 6 g* | *Prep time: 30 minutes* | *Cook time: 0 minutes*

PEANUT SAUCE
¼ cup all-natural peanut butter
1 tablespoon Homemade Hoisin Sauce (page 177)
1½ tablespoons reduced-sodium soy sauce
½ garlic clove, grated or minced

SPRING ROLLS
1 carrot, julienned
1 green onion, julienned
½ red bell pepper, julienned
¼ cup thinly sliced cabbage
1 tablespoon fresh lemon juice
1 teaspoon reduced-sodium soy sauce
2 tablespoons chopped fresh cilantro
8 (22-cm) rice paper rounds

1. Make the peanut sauce: In a small bowl, whisk together the peanut sauce ingredients and ¼ cup water until well combined. Set aside to let the flavors blend while you work on the spring rolls. You can do this 2 to 3 hours ahead of time if you like.

2. Make the spring rolls: In a medium bowl, toss together the carrot, green onion, bell pepper, cabbage, lemon juice, soy sauce, and cilantro.

3. Fill a pie pan with water, place a tea towel on a clean surface, and set out a plate to collect the finished spring rolls.

4. Following the directions on the packaging and working with one at a time, soak the rice paper rounds in the water for about 20 seconds to soften. When the rice paper is soft and flexible, gently spread it out on the tea towel. Add about ¼ cup of the veggie mixture to the center, fold the top and bottom over the veggies, overlapping the paper, fold over one side, and roll them up like a little burrito (the package might give instructions for this). Don't be intimidated—if you mess up, dump the veggies back into the bowl, return the rice paper round to the water, and start over. Place the finished spring roll on the plate and continue to make the rest (leave some space between them to prevent sticking).

5. Cover the spring rolls with plastic wrap and refrigerate for 15 to 30 minutes. Serve cold with the peanut sauce. Store leftover spring rolls in an airtight container in the refrigerator for up to 3 days.

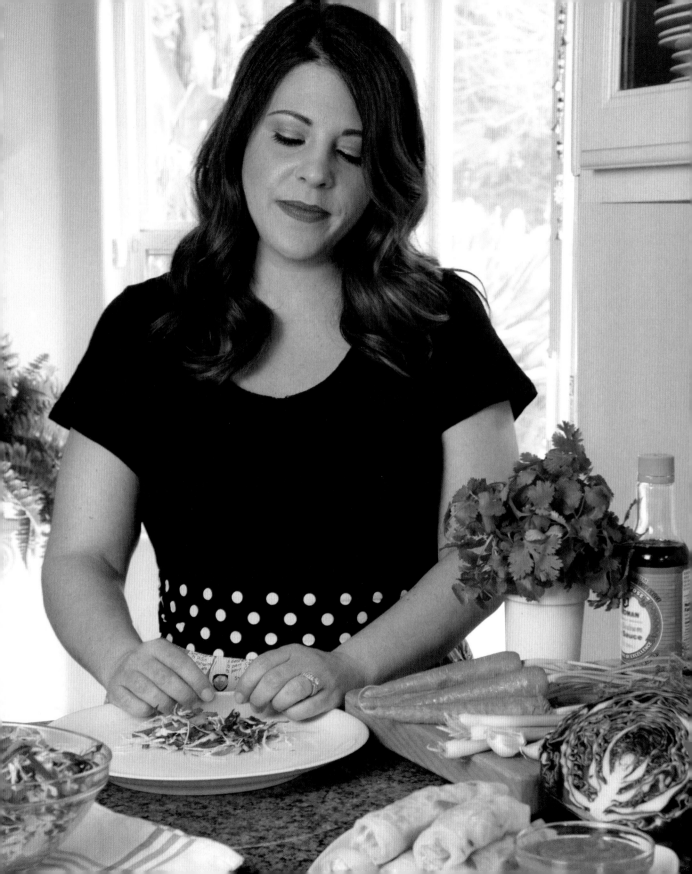

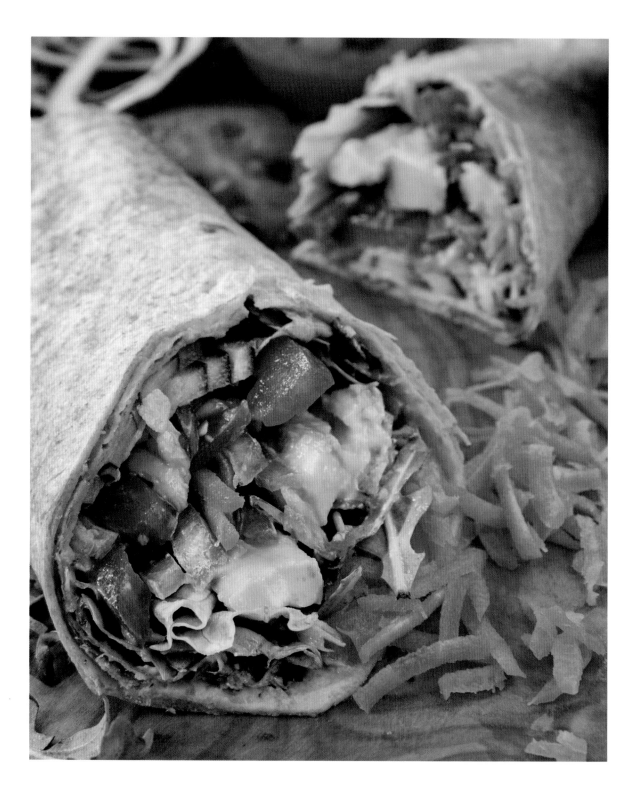

Farmers' Market Wrap

Oh, how I love this wrap! I must start by saying it's inspired by a sandwich created by Marcus Samuelsson. Marcus was my mentor on ABC's *The Taste*, and I'm pretty sure he would approve of this carb-cutting version. But do you want to know what I really love about it? It tastes great, of course—but those colors! It's like a rainbow of veggie beauty—a treat for the eyes as well as the taste buds. Try it—I know you'll love it!

Makes 1 serving | Serving size: 1 wrap | Per serving: calories 410; fat 23.5 g; saturated fat 7 g; fiber 11 g; protein 14 g; carbohydrates 39.5 g; sugar 7.5 g | Prep time: 10 minutes | Cook time: 0 minutes

1 (10-inch) burrito-size whole wheat tortilla
1 tablespoon Homemade Hummus (page 287)
½ carrot, grated
½ avocado, thinly sliced
¼ red bell pepper, cut into thin strips
2 red onion slices
2 tomato slices
¼ cup mixed greens
2 tablespoons shredded sharp cheddar cheese
2 tablespoons chopped fresh flat-leaf parsley

1. Place the tortilla on a clean surface, smear the hummus all over one side, and add the carrot, avocado, bell pepper, onion, tomato, and greens. Sprinkle with the cheese and top with the parsley.

2. Wrap up the tortilla like a sushi hand roll—where the bottom is narrow and the top wide—it will be kinda big and messy, but aren't all the best things in life? Get yourself a napkin (or two) and enjoy!

Chicken Salad Wraps

In my first cookbook, *Lose Weight by Eating*, I made a sweet-and-savory chicken salad with cranberries and pecans—yum! Like that recipe, this one uses Greek yogurt in place of mayo, cutting hundreds of calories while still giving you a creamy, flavorful chicken salad. Try this smart swap—I know you'll love it!

Makes 2 servings | *Serving size: 1 wrap* | *Per serving: calories 371; fat 8 g; saturated fat 4 g; fiber 28 g; protein 31 g; carbohydrates 40 g; sugar 6 g* | *Prep time: 15 minutes* | *Cook time: 0 minutes*

1 shredded cooked chicken breast
  (see page 132)
1 green onion, minced
½ red bell pepper, minced
1 small carrot, grated
¼ cup chopped fresh flat-leaf parsley
2 tablespoons shredded sharp cheddar cheese
½ cup 0% Greek yogurt
1 tablespoon Dijon mustard (or use your favorite
  mustard)
Kosher salt and freshly ground black pepper
2 burrito-size whole wheat wraps
1 cup mixed greens

1. In a medium bowl, mix together the chicken, green onion, bell pepper, carrot, parsley, cheese, yogurt, mustard, and a pinch each of salt and pepper until well combined. Taste for seasoning and add more salt and pepper as needed.

2. Place the wraps on a cutting board and top each with half the greens, then half the chicken salad, and roll up like a letter: Fold one-third over the middle third and the remaining third over that, overlapping in the center. Cut in half and enjoy.

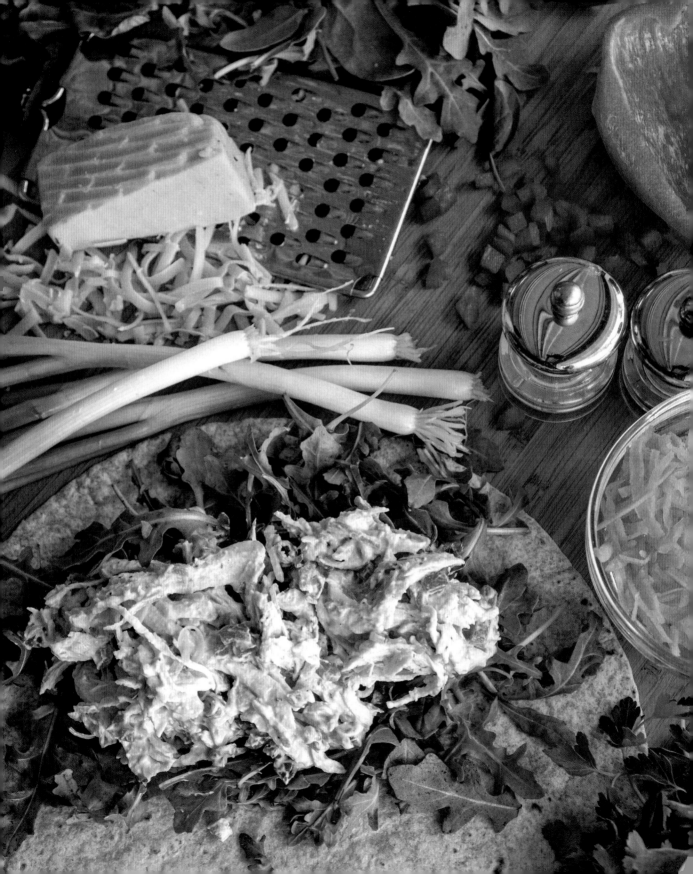

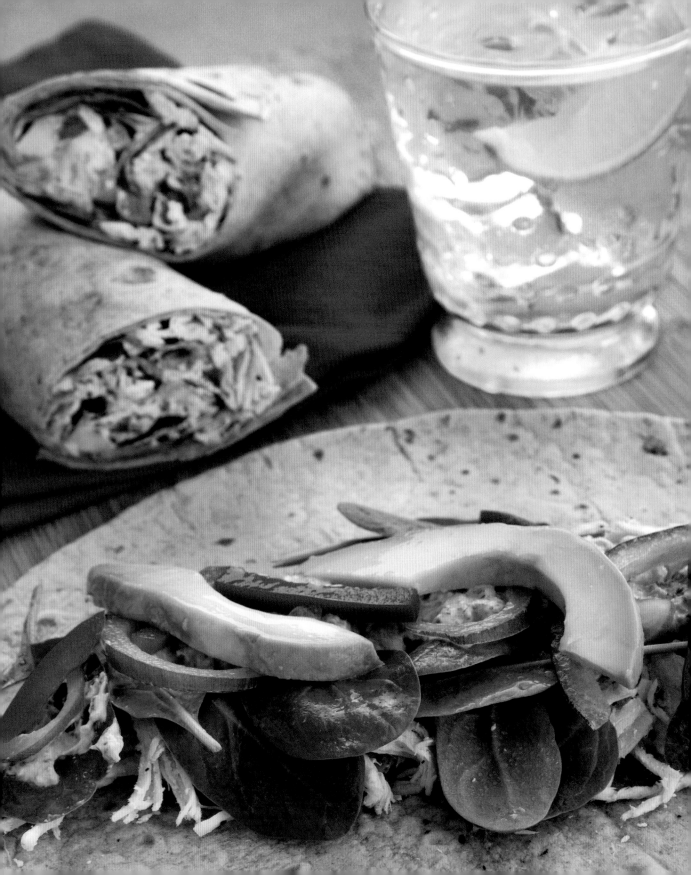

Chicken Avocado Wrap
with Creamy Pesto Sauce

I truly have a soft spot for the combo of pesto, avocado, and chicken! They go so well together that I find myself making all sorts of dishes with them, and this happens to be my current favorite—though the pesto chicken sandwiches in my first cookbook are perfectly divine.

Warning: This is a messy wrap but not too messy to bring with you in your lunch box. Just pack extra napkins!

You'll have plenty of extra pesto—try the Pesto Pea Soup on page 58!

Makes 2 servings | Serving size: 1 wrap | Per serving: calories 454; fat 20 g; saturated fat: 4 g; fiber 11 g; protein 24 g; carbohydrates 46 g; sugar 4 g | Prep time: 10 minutes | Cook time: 0 minutes

SKINNY PESTO

1 cup fresh basil leaves

1 tablespoon olive oil

2 tablespoons slivered almonds

1 garlic clove

1 tablespoon freshly shredded Parmesan cheese

WRAPS

⅓ cup 0% Greek yogurt

1 cooked boneless, skinless chicken breast (see page 132)

2 (10-inch) burrito-size spinach or whole wheat wraps

½ cup spinach

1 avocado, thinly sliced

½ red bell pepper, sliced into strips

2 red onion slices

1. Make the pesto: Place all the ingredients in a food processor and process until smooth. Transfer to a jar, tightly cover, and store in the fridge for up to 1 week.

2. Make the wraps: In a small bowl, mix together 2 tablespoons of the pesto with the yogurt until well combined.

3. Slice the chicken into strips and place them in the middle of each wrap. Top with the spinach, the pesto-yogurt mixture, the avocado, bell pepper, and onion. Roll up the wraps like a burrito, cut them in half, and dig in.

Butternut Squash Wrap

This one is a shout-out to all my Instagram pals! I posted photos of this recipe while I was testing it and people went nuts. Sorry to make you all wait—but it will be worth it!

Butternut squash is by far my favorite squash; it's packed full of dietary fiber and potassium, making it a wonderful before- or after-workout meal. It's also great for your immune system, helping bolster you during cold and flu season. I like to cube my butternut squash and freeze it so it's ready to go when I need it. A little prep work after grocery shopping will set you up for the whole week.

If you're planning on taking these wraps in your lunch box, you can roast the squash ahead of time, refrigerate, then throw it together in the morning.

Makes 2 servings | Serving size: 1 wrap | Per serving: calories 355; fat 13 g; saturated fat 3.5 g; fiber 31 g; protein 13 g; carbohydrates 49 g; sugar 6 g | Prep time: 20 minutes | Cook time: 35 minutes

²/₃ cup ½-inch-cubed butternut squash
1 teaspoon olive oil
2 tablespoons 0% Greek yogurt
2 teaspoons Dijon mustard
2 (8-inch) whole wheat tortillas
2 small carrots, grated (use purple carrots if you can get them—so pretty!)
2 Persian cucumbers or 1 (4-inch) piece cucumber, thinly sliced
½ avocado, sliced
²/₃ cup arugula

1. Preheat the oven to 375°F.

2. In a 9 × 9-inch casserole dish, toss the butternut squash in the oil to coat. Spread the squash in a single layer and roast for 35 minutes, or until soft.

3. In a small bowl, mix together the yogurt and mustard. Set aside.

4. Let the squash cool for 5 minutes before handling. If you're making this wrap for a lunch box, cover the ingredients and refrigerate them for fast prep later in the week.

5. To assemble the wraps, smear each tortilla with the yogurt-mustard spread, then top with the carrots, cucumbers, avocado, and arugula. Wrap like you're folding a letter—fold one third over the middle and the remaining third over that, overlapping in the center—and cut in half. They'll be big and messy—you'll need several napkins . . . and maybe a bib.

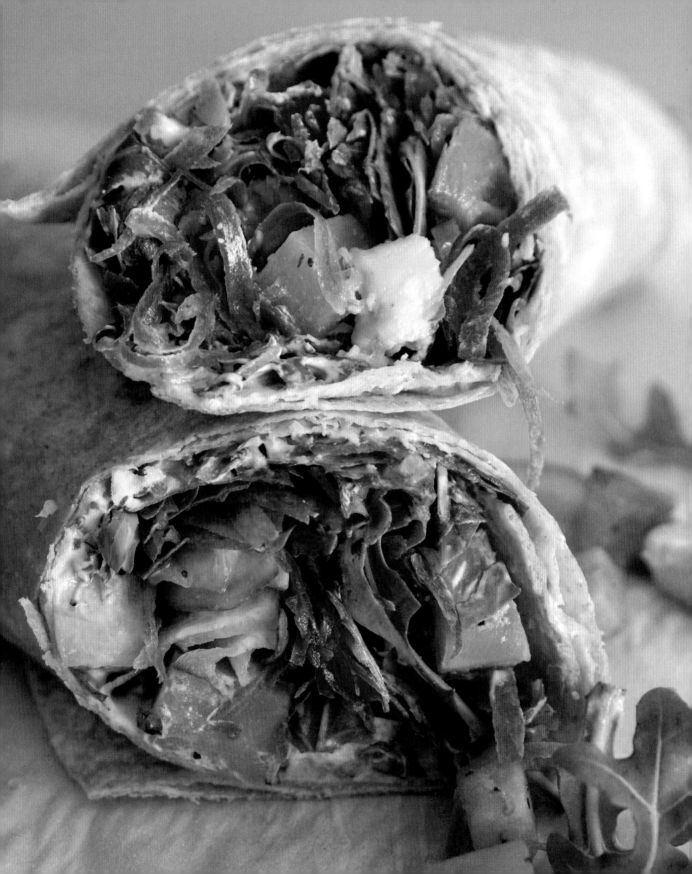

Caesar Salad Wrap with Creamy Dip

These super-simple wraps are so satisfying! They also travel well, making them great for lunch boxes.

If you have some leftover cooked chicken, use it up here and save yourself some time and money!

Makes 2 servings | Serving size: 1 wrap | Per serving: calories 476; fat 20 g; saturated fat 5 g; fiber 8 g; protein 29 g; carbohydrates 46 g; sugar 6 g | Prep time: 5 minutes | Cook time: 12 minutes

DIP
1 tablespoon fresh lemon juice
1½ teaspoons Dijon mustard
½ cup 0% Greek yogurt
1 tablespoon balsamic vinegar
1 garlic clove

WRAP
1 boneless, skinless chicken breast
1 teaspoon extra-virgin olive oil
Pinch of garlic salt
2 (10-inch) burrito-size spinach wraps (they look like green tortillas; you'll find them by the tortillas or bread)
4 large romaine leaves
2 tablespoons freshly grated Parmesan cheese
1 avocado, sliced (optional)

1. Make the dip: In a small bowl, combine the lemon juice, mustard, yogurt, and vinegar. Use a fine grater to shred the garlic clove into the bowl, just to the point where you are worried you might cut yourself (so about two-thirds of the clove), and discard the rest. Mix well and set aside to marinate.

2. Make the wrap: Coat the chicken breast with oil and a pinch of garlic salt. Heat a small skillet over medium-high heat and add the chicken. Cover and cook for 4 to 6 minutes per side, until cooked through (no pink on the inside and the juices run clear). Transfer the chicken to a plate to cool, then shred it with two forks.

3. Place the spinach wraps on a clean surface (or on parchment paper, if you're wrapping them to go) and layer the romaine leaves over the wraps. Top with the chicken, Parmesan, and avocado (if using).

4. Roll up the wraps like you are folding a letter: fold one-third over the middle third and the remaining third over that, overlapping in the center. Place them seam side down on a plate and slice the wraps in half. Divide the dip between two small ramekins if you're eating them now, or place the wraps and dip in separate containers to enjoy later. Dip the wraps, then devour them!

7

Salads Masquerading as Hot Meals

Hurray—the healthy qualities of a veggie-loaded salad with the pleasure of a hot meal! From soups to stir-fry to hearty chili, here are some ways to get your salad fix without a bit of cold crunch—perfect for chilly days and skeptical family members.

Use these for any of your detox salads—they're packed full of greens and will help speed up your metabolism while filling you up.

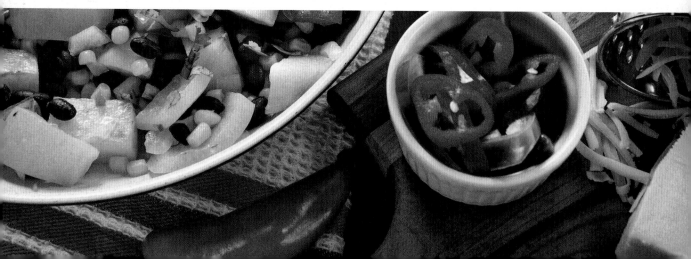

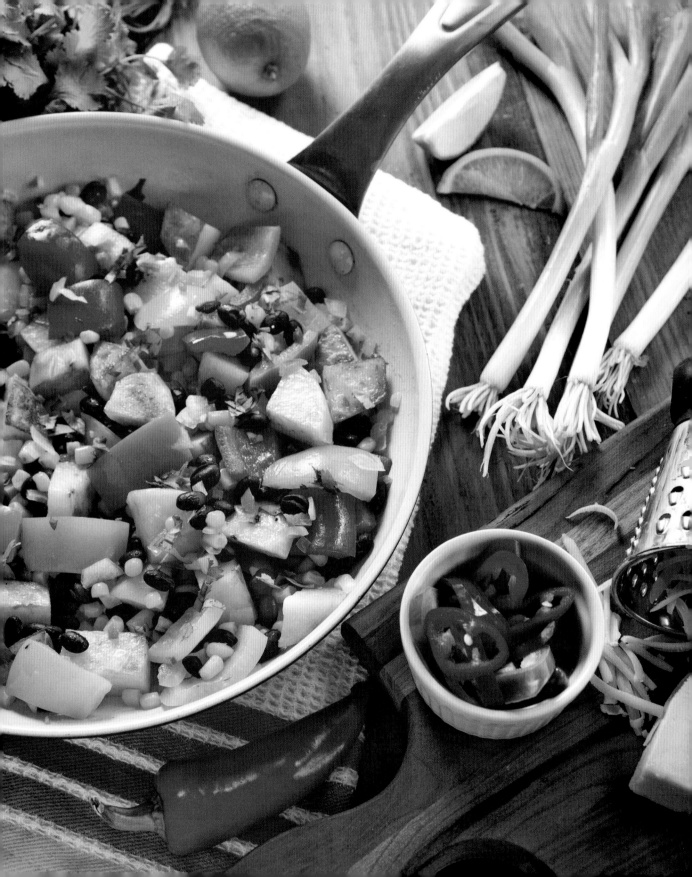

Veggie Skillet with Topping Bar

This has been one of my favorite cold-day lunch go-tos for years, and yes, it's on the blog. But here I've added a topping bar to make it new and fresh. I eventually started making this skillet as a side dish with dinner (which I highly recommend), and that's where the topping bar came in—serve the family a ton of veggies and they may not be too thrilled about it, but let them top it with all their favorite goodies and they'll ask for it again and again!

Makes 2 servings | Serving size: about 2½ cups | Per serving: calories 350; fat 6 g; saturated fat 1 g; fiber 12 g; protein 11 g; carbohydrates 68 g; sugar 11 g | Prep time: 20 minutes | Cook time: 35 minutes

2 teaspoons olive oil

2 medium Yukon Gold potatoes, cut into bite-size cubes

2 red bell peppers, cut into bite-size chunks

1 jalapeño, ribs and seeds removed, chopped

1 medium white or yellow onion, chopped

1 garlic clove, chopped

Pinch of salt

Fresh corn kernels from 1 large ear, or ½ cup frozen corn, thawed

½ cup canned black beans, drained and rinsed

1 tablespoon fresh lime juice

¼ cup chopped fresh cilantro (if you don't like cilantro, use flat-leaf parsley)

TOPPING BAR (ALL OPTIONAL)

Greek yogurt (tastes like sour cream!)

More chopped fresh cilantro

Lime wedges

Shredded sharp cheddar cheese

Rings of fresh or pickled jalapeño

Sliced green onions

Hot sauce or salsa

Sliced avocado

1. Heat 1 teaspoon of the oil in a large skillet over medium heat. Add the potatoes, cover, and cook for about 20 minutes, until soft, stirring two or three times to avoid burning.

2. Add the bell peppers, jalapeño, onion, and garlic, drizzle the remaining 1 teaspoon oil on top, and stir. Add the salt and cook for 10 minutes, uncovered, stirring occasionally to avoid burning.

3. Add the corn, beans, and lime juice and cook for 5 minutes to warm them. Top with the cilantro and serve right out of the hot skillet (or plate it if you have kids) with any or all of the toppings on the side.

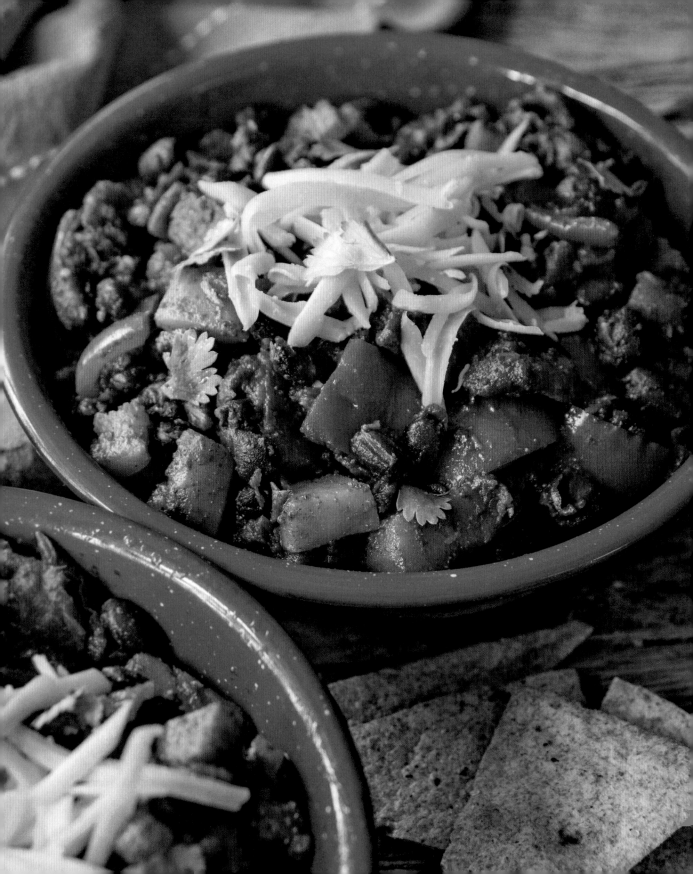

Butternut Squash Chili

Oh man, the first day I made this I yelled out (to an empty house, mind you), "Holy crap, this is good!" I've made a lot of chili in my life, as you well know if you follow my blog, but this one is my current favorite. I could eat it every day for lunch and be a happy camper.

This amazing-tasting chili is also great for you. It's naturally metabolism boosting, and—my personal favorite—it's packed full of beautifying ingredients. Chili that makes you pretty—love it!

Makes 2 servings | Serving size: 1¼ cups | Per serving: calories 120; fat 1 g; saturated fat 0.5 g; fiber 6 g; protein 15 g; carbohydrates 24 g; sugar 9 g | Prep time: 15 minutes | Cook time: 60 minutes

1 teaspoon olive oil
2 cups ½-inch-cubed butternut squash
1 medium red onion, cut into ½-inch dice
1 red bell pepper, cut into ½-inch dice
Pinch of kosher salt
4 garlic cloves, chopped
10 large tomatoes, chopped
2 (15-ounce) cans black beans, drained and
    rinsed (preferably BPA-free cans)
2 bay leaves
3 tablespoons chili powder
1 teaspoon ground cumin
¼ teaspoon ground nutmeg
1 cup vegetable or bone broth
Dash of hot sauce (optional)

OPTIONAL TOPPINGS
0% Greek yogurt
Hot sauce
Chopped fresh cilantro
Sliced green onions
Crumbled tortilla chips (see page 278)
Grated sharp cheddar cheese

1. Heat the oil in a large saucepan over medium heat. Add the squash, onion, bell pepper, and salt. Cook, stirring often, until the veggies begin to soften, about 10 minutes.

2. Add the garlic and tomatoes and cook for about 5 minutes, until the tomatoes start to break down. Add the beans, bay leaves, chili powder, cumin, nutmeg, broth, and hot sauce (if using) and stir to combine. Cover and cook on medium-low heat for about 45 minutes, until the liquid has reduced, stirring a few times to avoid burning.

3. Remove and discard the bay leaves and serve with any or all of the optional toppings. I love this with just yogurt, cilantro, and more hot sauce!

Ratatouille

I just love that this wonderful French peasant dish has become well-known thanks to Disney and the hilarious voice of Patton Oswalt! But for those of you who have not heard of this amazing dish, let me explain. It's simply a thick vegetable stew with a tomato base, it's elegant and simple, and best of all, it originated in Nice, France . . . isn't that nice? The more traditional ratatouille recipes call for you to cook each vegetable individually, but I wanted to make this as simple as possible, so to the purists, please forgive me! It's just a chop-and-dump kind of meal, keeping it easy for new and busy cooks. While each veggie is cooking, simply cut up the next one. There's about 10 minutes between cooking each vegetable, giving you plenty of downtime to prep.

Makes 2 servings | Per serving: calories 137; fat 7.5 g; saturated fat 1 g; fiber 4 g; protein 3 g; carbohydrates 17 g; sugar 9 g | Prep time: 25 minutes | Cook time: 1 hour 5 minutes

3 teaspoons olive oil
1 medium white or yellow onion
Kosher salt
1 red bell pepper
1 medium eggplant
1 zucchini
3 plum tomatoes
3 garlic cloves
½ cup chopped fresh basil
Leaves from 2 thyme sprigs
1 teaspoon red wine vinegar
Freshly ground black pepper

1. In a Dutch oven or large saucepan over medium heat, heat ¾ teaspoon of the oil. Slice the onion and add it to the pan with a pinch of salt. Sauté for 10 minutes, or until tender.

2. Cut the bell peppers into bite-size chunks. Add another ¾ teaspoon of the oil to the pan, then the bell pepper. Toss to coat and sauté for 10 minutes, or until tender.

3. Leaving the skin on, cut the eggplant into ½-inch cubes. Add another ¾ teaspoon of the oil to the pan, then the eggplant. Toss and sauté for 10 minutes, or until tender.

4. Slice the zucchini into ½-inch-thick rings. Add the remaining ¾ teaspoon oil, then the zucchini. Toss and sauté for 10 minutes, or until tender.

5. Chop the tomatoes into ½-inch chunks and add them to the pan. Cook for 5 minutes, then add the basil and thyme. Cover and cook for 20 minutes, or until soft. Stir in the vinegar and pepper to taste and serve.

6. This dish can be made ahead and reheated in the oven at 350°F for 30 minutes. It's also good room temperature and even cold, right out of the fridge.

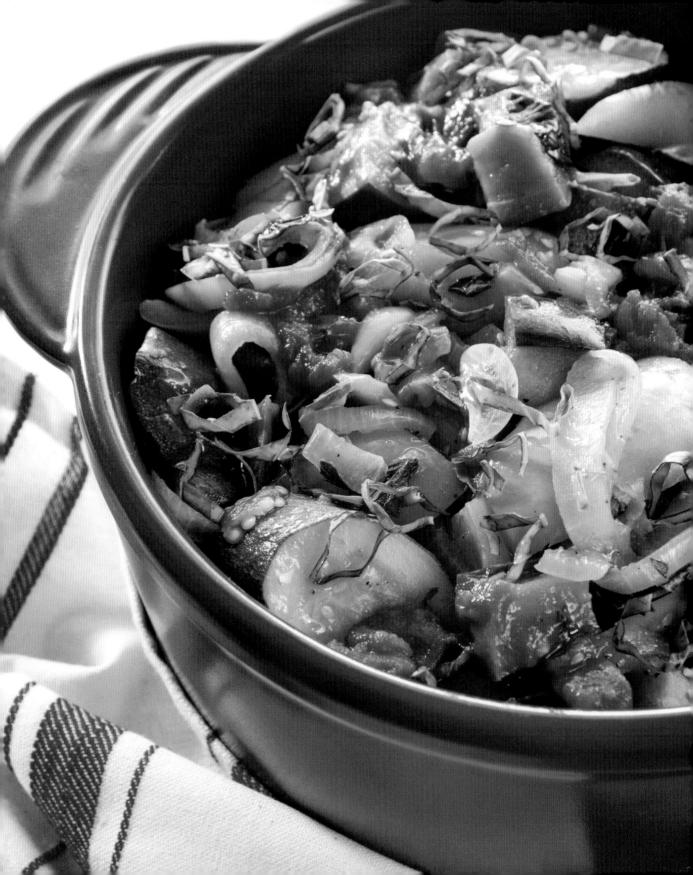

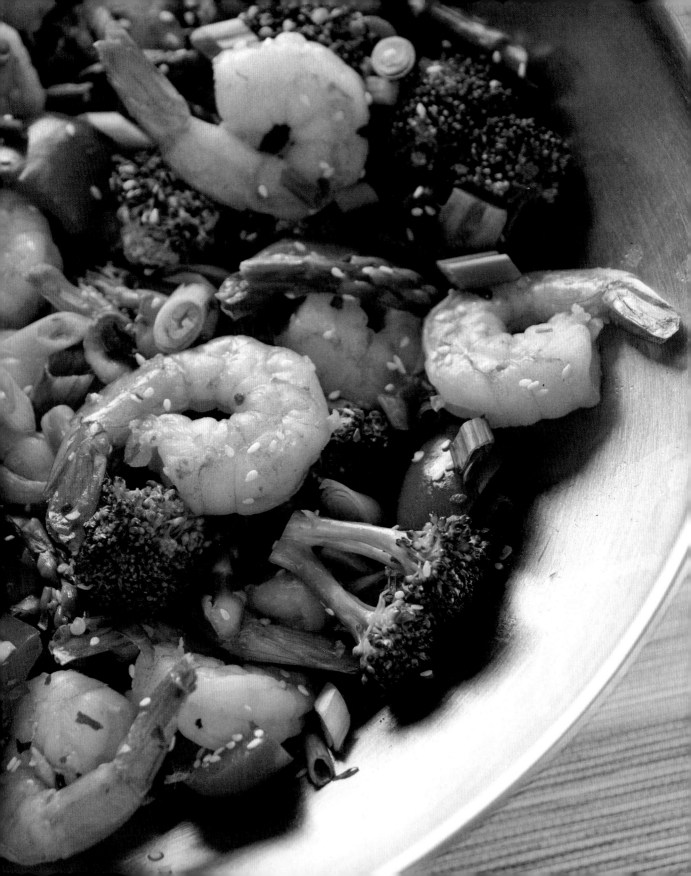

Shrimp Stir-Fry

As far as "cooked salads" go, I'd have to say this is one of the best! It's so hearty and filling and a great way to get your veggies in on a cold rainy day, or any day for that matter. Swap the shrimp for cubed chicken if you prefer. Vegans and vegetarians, add 2 cups of cubed tofu in place of the shrimp.

Makes 4 servings | *Serving size: about 2 cups* | *Per serving: calories 214; fat 7 g; saturated fat 1 g; fiber 5 g; protein 28 g; carbohydrates 11.5 g; sugar 4.5 g* | *Prep time: 10 minutes* | *Cook time: 20 minutes*

1 pound extra-large shrimp, peeled and deveined
1 tablespoon toasted sesame oil
2 garlic cloves, minced
1 teaspoon red pepper flakes
2 cups sliced white mushrooms
1 bunch asparagus, trimmed and cut into bite-size pieces (about 3 cups)
1 red bell pepper, cut into bite-size pieces
2 cups broccoli florets
1 tablespoon reduced-sodium soy sauce
1 teaspoon fish sauce
1 teaspoon sriracha (optional)
1 tablespoon sesame seeds
2 green onions, sliced on the diagonal

1. In a medium bowl, toss together the shrimp, ½ tablespoon of the oil, and half the garlic until well coated. Set aside to marinate while you chop the vegetables.

2. Heat a large sauté pan over medium heat. Add the shrimp and cook for about 1 minute on each side, until lightly browned. Transfer the shrimp to a plate.

3. Add the remaining ½ tablespoon oil and the red pepper flakes to the sauté pan, then add the mushrooms, asparagus, bell pepper, broccoli, and remaining garlic. Stir to combine, then cook for about 5 minutes, until the vegetables are tender, stirring often to avoid burning. Stir in the soy sauce, fish sauce, and sriracha and cook for about 10 minutes, until the vegetables start to soften.

4. Return the shrimp to the sauté pan, add the sesame seeds, and toss together with the vegetables. Cook for 1 to 3 minutes, until the shrimp is fully cooked and pink. Plate and top with the green onions.

Broccoli Parmesan

When I was growing up, this was the only way my mother could get my step-father to eat any greens—cover broccoli with homemade marinara sauce and cheese. It's so delicious and so much easier than making lasagna—and no carb-laden pasta!

This dish travels very well, so bring it to potlucks or portion out individual servings and take in your lunch box.

Makes 3 servings | Serving size: 2 cups | Per serving: calories 217; fat 9.5 g; saturated fat 3.5 g; fiber 8 g; protein 13 g; carbohydrates 26 g; sugar 10 g | Prep time: 10 minutes | Cook time: 50 minutes

6 cups broccoli florets
2 teaspoons olive oil
1½ cups marinara sauce (see page 155)
½ cup shredded mozzarella
2 tablespoons freshly grated Parmesan cheese

1. Preheat the oven to 350°F.

2. Place the broccoli in a 9 × 13-inch baking dish, toss with the oil, and roast for 40 minutes, stirring twice to avoid burning.

3. Pull the baking dish from the oven, stir the broccoli, and top with the marinara sauce, mozzarella, and Parmesan. Return to the oven for about 10 minutes, until the cheese is melted and golden on the edges. That's it—so easy! Move leftovers to individual-size storage containers for homemade frozen meals.

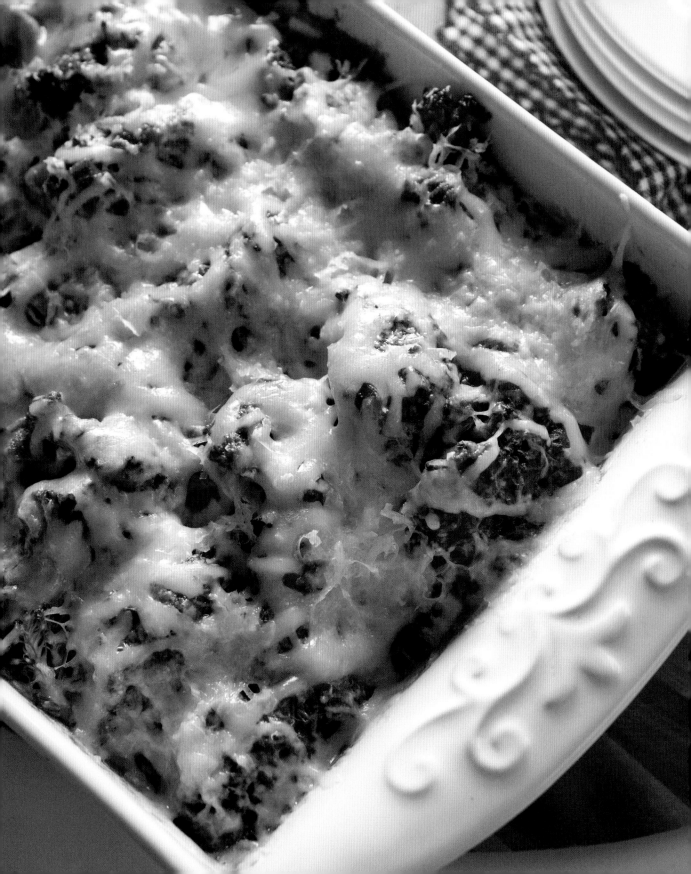

Black Bean "Enchilada" Spaghetti Squash

My neighbors grow their own spaghetti squash, so guess who's the lucky recipient at harvest season? That's right, *me!*

Originally I was going to make a pasta-like dish here, but that is so played out. So often people go right to making an Italian dish with spaghetti squash, but I went another route, smothering the squash with fresh enchilada sauce and cheese and making something new and exciting with this pasta-like veggie! You're welcome.

Makes 2 servings | Serving size: ½ spaghetti squash (about 2½ cups) | Per serving: calories 446; fat 15 g; saturated fat 6.5 g; fiber 17.5 g; protein 22 g; carbohydrates 59 g; sugar 14.5 g
Prep time: 15 minutes | Cook time: 1 hour 30 minutes

1 (4-pound) spaghetti squash, halved and seeded
Olive oil spray
5 large tomatoes, cored and quartered
1 jalapeño, ribs and seeds removed, diced
1 medium yellow onion, diced
1 garlic clove, quartered
½ teaspoon fresh thyme or ¼ teaspoon dried
Pinch of kosher salt
½ teaspoon ground allspice
1 teaspoon garlic powder
¼ teaspoon freshly ground black pepper
1 (15-ounce) can black beans, drained and rinsed (preferably BPA-free cans)
½ cup grated sharp cheddar cheese

OPTIONAL TOPPINGS
Chopped fresh cilantro
Sliced green onions
Hot sauce or salsa
0% Greek yogurt
Diced avocado

1. Preheat the oven to 375°F.

2. Spray the cut sides of the squash with oil spray and place the halves cut side down on a rimmed baking sheet. Roast for about 1 hour; the squash is done when you push on the outside with a wooden spoon and it's no longer hard as a rock (technical, I know).

3. Meanwhile, spray a large skillet with oil spray and place over medium heat. Add the tomatoes, jalapeño, onion, garlic, thyme, and salt, then cover and sauté until the onion and jalapeño are very soft, 10 to 15 minutes.

4. Transfer the veggies to a blender and add 1 cup water, the allspice, garlic powder, and pepper. Blend, with the top lightly vented, until smooth.

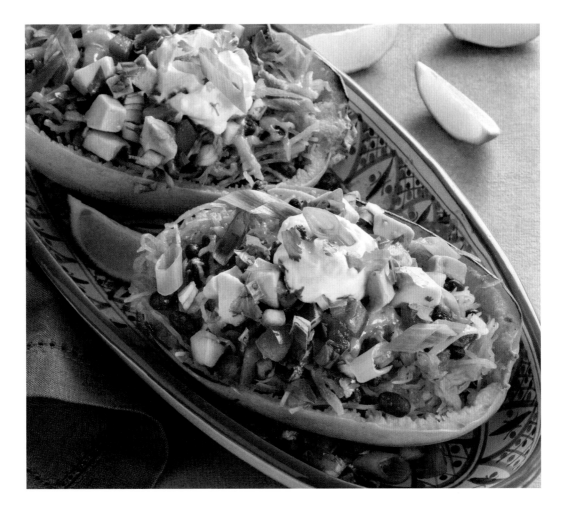

5. Transfer the sauce back to the original skillet and simmer until reduced and thickened, about 10 minutes. Leave a couple tablespoons of the sauce in the skillet and transfer the rest to a medium bowl and set aside.

6. When the squash is done, remove it from the oven but leave the oven on. Carefully (with oven mitts on!) flip over the squash halves to expose the insides, then set aside to cool for about 10 minutes. Shred the squash flesh with a fork and add it to the skillet with the sauce (reserve the empty squash skins).

7. Add the beans to the skillet and toss to combine with the squash. Spoon the mixture back into the squash skins, then top with the reserved sauce and cheese.

8. Return to the oven for 25 minutes, or until the cheese is melted and the filling is bubbling. Garnish with the desired toppings and dig in!

Overloaded Baked Potato

Hello from Idaho, land of potatoes! Halfway through writing this book, I moved to Boise, and as a potato lover, I was thrilled at the abundance of locally grown, inexpensive potatoes. Even organic potatoes are pretty inexpensive, a great boost for those of us on a budget.

Now, some of you might be scratching your heads and thinking, *Potatoes are bad for you—starch and carbs cause weight gain*, so let's talk about that for a minute. A medium potato has only about 160 calories, is packed full of fiber and potassium, and contains (you may want to sit down for this) 70 percent of your daily recommended vitamin C! Translation: Potatoes are great for staying full, building lean muscle, and, best of all, boosting your metabolism (thanks to the vitamin C). Compare that to another starchy carbohydrate, such as rice. For the same serving, you're looking at more than 200 calories, more carbohydrates, less-filling fiber, and practically no vitamins. So here's a very healthy alternative when you're craving carbs or starchy foods.

Makes 2 servings | Serving size: 2 potato halves | Per serving: calories 488; fat 15 g; saturated fat 7 g; fiber 8 g; protein 41 g; carbohydrates 50 g; sugar 7.5 g | Prep time: 10 minutes | Cook time: 1 hour 30 minutes

2 medium russet potatoes

1 tablespoon olive oil

2 boneless, skinless chicken breasts, cut into ¼-inch cubes

Kosher salt

1 red bell pepper, cut into thin strips

½ medium red onion, chopped

1 cup broccoli florets

1 cup sliced white mushrooms

½ cup chopped zucchini

1 to 2 teaspoons red pepper flakes (depending on your heat preference)

2 garlic cloves, minced

Juice from ½ lime

½ cup grated cheddar cheese

2 tablespoons minced fresh flat-leaf parsley

⅓ cup 0% Greek yogurt (optional)

Hot sauce (optional)

1. Preheat the oven to 350°F.

2. Stab the potatoes a few times all over with a fork, place them on the bottom oven rack, and bake for 1 hour.

3. Meanwhile, in a large sauté pan, heat ½ tablespoon of the oil over medium-high heat. Add the chicken cubes and toss to coat in oil. Cook for about 5 minutes, until lightly browned (the chicken will not be done cooking yet), and transfer to a plate.

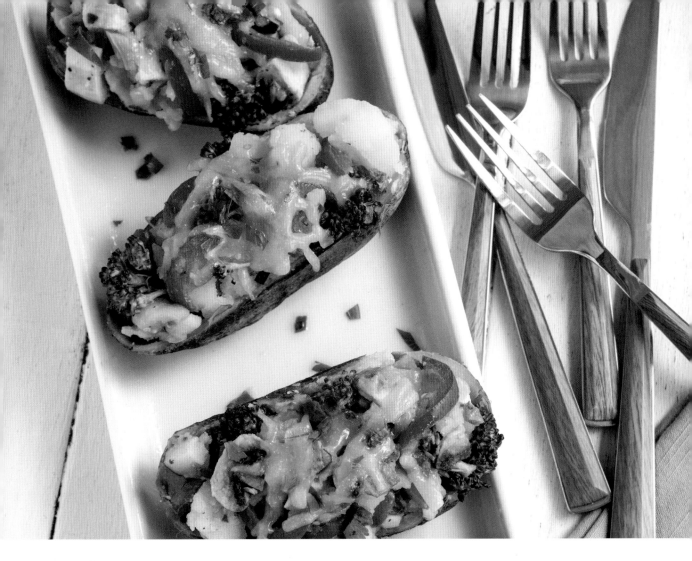

4. Add the remaining ½ tablespoon oil, the bell pepper, onion, broccoli, mushrooms, and zucchini and sauté for about 5 minutes, until they start to sweat, then add the red pepper flakes, garlic, and lime juice. Continue sautéing for another 5 minutes, or until the veggies start to soften. Add the chicken and any juices from the plate and cook for 5 minutes more, or until the chicken is cooked through.

5. When the potatoes are cool enough to handle, cut them in half lengthwise and use a spoon to scoop the flesh into the sauté pan, leaving the skins intact. Smash the potato flesh with a wooden spoon and mix it with the rest of the filling.

6. Place the potato skins on a baking sheet and divide the filling among the four potato skins, letting it mound so that you use all the filling.

7. Top with the cheese and bake for 5 minutes, or until the cheese is melted and bubbling. Sprinkle with the parsley and (if using) top with both the yogurt and hot sauce. Serve hot and enjoy.

Loaded Broccoli Potato Soup

Here's a cross between a creamy broccoli soup and loaded potato soup, and to be frank, it tastes mostly like a potato soup with pretty little green flecks in it.

I've suggested lots of fun toppings; choose what you like, and if you're looking for a vegan soup, simply swap out the butter and cheese for your favorite vegan substitutes. You really can't hurt this soup—it's resilient!

Makes 6 servings | Serving size: 1 cup | Per serving: calories 205; fat 5 g; saturated fat 2 g; fiber 4 g; protein 5.5 g; carbohydrates 34 g; sugar 7 g | Prep time: 15 minutes | Cook time: 60 minutes

1 tablespoon unsalted butter
1 medium yellow onion, roughly chopped
3 garlic cloves, chopped
1 tablespoon all-purpose flour
3 cups vegetable broth
3 cups unsweetened almond milk
4 medium russet potatoes, peeled and cut into
    ½-inch dice
1 cup roughly chopped broccoli
¼ cup grated sharp cheddar cheese
Kosher salt and freshly ground black pepper

OPTIONAL TOPPINGS
Grated sharp cheddar cheese
0% Greek yogurt
Diced cooked turkey bacon
Green onions, sliced on the diagonal
Hot sauce

1. In a large saucepan, melt the butter over medium heat. Add the onion and sauté until it starts to turn translucent, about 10 minutes. Add the garlic and cook for about 1 minute, until it softens, then add the flour and mix until a paste starts to form.

2. Add ½ cup of the broth and whisk together well, then add the remaining 2½ cups broth and the almond milk. Add the potatoes and broccoli and cook for about 20 minutes, until the potatoes are soft when pierced with a fork.

3. Turn off the heat and puree with an immersion blender until creamy (or use a traditional blender, but be sure to vent the top to avoid an explosion of hot soup).

4. Add the cheese, turn the heat to medium, and simmer for about 20 minutes, until slightly thickened. Season with salt and pepper (add salt judiciously if you're planning on topping with extra cheese and turkey bacon).

5. I like to serve this soup with a topping bar, and I simply must add cheese, yogurt, turkey bacon, and lots of green onions to my serving. Choose what you love and let the rest of the family do the same—they'll be more likely to love the meal if they make it their own.

Photo on page 57.

Italian Wedding Soup with Turkey Meatballs

I simply must make this soup with alphabet pasta; it's the way my mom made it. You can use any small pasta, but use whole wheat pasta if you can.

For my vegetarian friends, use vegetable broth in place of chicken broth, and just skip the meatballs. It's still a divine soup!

Makes 10 servings | Serving size: about 1¼ cups | Per serving: calories 159; fat 5.5 g; saturated fat 1 g; fiber 1 g; protein 15 g; carbohydrates 12 g; sugar 3 g | Prep time: 30 minutes | Cook time: 40 minutes

MEATBALLS
Olive oil spray
1 pound lean ground turkey
1 large egg
1 tablespoon freshly grated Parmesan cheese
3 tablespoons bread crumbs
1 garlic clove, minced
⅛ teaspoon kosher salt
⅛ teaspoon freshly ground black pepper

SOUP
Olive oil spray
1 medium yellow onion, minced
3 carrots, minced
2 celery stalks, minced
10 cups (2½ quarts) chicken broth
½ cup uncooked small whole wheat pasta (such as alphabet, stars, or orzo)
3 cups baby spinach

Grated Parmesan cheese, for serving (optional)

1. Make the meatballs: Preheat the oven to 350°F and spray a rimmed baking sheet with oil spray.

2. In a large bowl, combine the turkey, egg, cheese, bread crumbs, garlic, salt, and pepper. Using clean hands, mix together, then roll the mixture into 25 to 30 small meatballs, placing them on the prepared baking sheet as you work. Bake the meatballs for 30 minutes, or until cooked through.

3. Make the soup: Lightly spray a large saucepan with oil spray and heat over medium-high heat. Add the onion, carrots, and celery and cook for about 8 minutes, until the vegetables are soft.

4. Add the broth and bring to a boil. Add the pasta and the cooked meatballs and cook for 8 minutes, or until the pasta is cooked through.

5. To serve, add ⅓ cup of the baby spinach to a bowl and top with 1¼ cups of the soup. Sprinkle on a little more Parmesan if you like, and enjoy. Let the leftovers cool, then move them to a freezer bag and freeze for up to 3 months

Photo on page 57.

8

No-Cook Detox Meals

One of the biggest requests for this book was no-cook meals, and with this chapter, along with chapters 2, and 4, you'll have an abundance of meals that barely require a kitchen.

These meals are great for lunches and dinners, and you can use them as detox meals for all the detox plans. Most of them can be tossed together in a manner of moments, others will give you leftovers, and others (like the ceviche) won't require cooking but will require time.

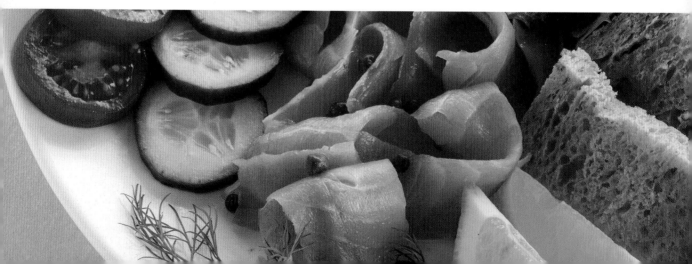

*Okay, okay . . . some of these recipes do require light cooking, but they are super simple, won't require much cook time, and can easily be made ahead.

Healthy "Lunchables"

I truly hate to knock a food that basically sustained my life during the nineties, but with processed meat and cheese, crackers packed with preservatives and chemicals, and lots of salt and fat, they're just not healthy. But because the lovely people at Lunchables fed me through my school years, I figured I would use them as my muse in this recipe and try not to talk too much crap.

Because Lunchables come in many combinations, I've given you three. Even though a couple of these do require a little cook time, they're great make-ahead lunches, so get yourself a few food-storage containers with separate compartments and pack a week's worth to grab and go.

Makes 1 to 3 servings, depending on how many combinations you choose to make
Serving size: 1 "Lunchable" | Prep time: about 15 minutes each | Cook time: 0 to 30 minutes

Classic Style
(a very loose definition . . . basically this is a stackable meal)

Per serving: calories 497; fat 34 g; saturated fat 3.5 g; fiber 8.5 g; protein 23 g; carbohydrates 39 g; sugar 18 g

1 boneless, skinless chicken breast
½ teaspoon olive oil
Kosher salt and freshly ground black pepper
2 ounces sharp cheddar cheese, thinly sliced
½ cucumber, cut into ¼-inch-thick slices
¼ cup Homemade Hummus (page 287)

1. Brush the chicken breast with the oil and sprinkle it lightly with salt and pepper. Heat a small skillet over medium-high heat and cook the chicken, covered, for 4 to 6 minutes on each side, until cooked through (no pink on the inside and the juices run clear). Let it cool for 5 minutes, then cut it into thin slices.

2. Place the chicken, cheese, and cucumber slices in separate compartments of a food-storage container. Place the hummus in a small bowl or a dressing cup with a tight-fitting cover and close it all up. Store in the refrigerator for up to 3 days.

Vegan
Style

Classic
Style

Super-Easy
No-Cook Style

Vegan Style

(you know I love you, all my vegan and vegetarian friends)

Per serving: calories 492 g; fat 34 g; saturated fat 3.5 g; fiber 8.5 g; protein 23 g; carbohydrates 39 g; sugar 18 g

6 ounces extra-firm tofu
1 teaspoon chili powder
2 teaspoons garlic powder
1 teaspoon paprika
⅛ teaspoon kosher salt
⅛ teaspoon freshly ground black pepper
Olive oil spray
1 apple, cored and sliced
1 teaspoon lemon juice
2 carrots, cut into 2-inch sticks
2 tablespoons almond butter

1. Wrap the tofu in a clean tea towel and place it under a heavy object, such as a cast-iron skillet, for 30 minutes to draw out some of the moisture.

2. Meanwhile, in a small bowl, mix together the chili powder, garlic powder, paprika, salt, pepper, and 2 tablespoons water. Set aside.

3. Unwrap the tofu and cut it into ¼-inch-thick slices. Place it in a gallon-size freezer bag with the marinade, put it in the fridge, and let it soak up the flavors for at least 1 hour and up to overnight (the longer, the better).

4. Preheat the oven to 450°F.

5. Line a baking sheet with parchment paper, spray it with oil spray, and spread out the tofu on the sheet, reserving half the marinade. Bake for 15 minutes, flip, and spoon over half the marinade. Bake for 10 minutes, flip, add the rest of the marinade, and bake for another 5 minutes. Let the tofu cool for 5 minutes, then place it in one of the compartments of a food-storage container.

6. Toss the apple in the lemon juice to keep it from turning brown and place the carrots and apple in the remaining compartments. Place the almond butter in a small bowl or a dressing cup with a tight-fitting cover and close it all up. Store in the refrigerator for up to 3 days.

Photo on page 133.

Super-Easy No-Cook Style

(because life gets busy!)

Per serving: calories 370 g; fat 24 g; saturated fat 12 g; fiber 2 g; protein 37 g; carbohydrates 4 g; sugar 0 g

4 ounces premium-quality deli roast beef
2 ounces pepper Jack cheese (two slices pre-cut deli cheese), cut into small squares
2 endive heads, leaves separated, or 4 halved romaine leaves
¼ cup cherry tomatoes

Place the roast beef, cheese, greens, and tomatoes in separate compartments of a food-storage container. Optional add-ins, such as the pesto on page 107 or Homemade Hummus on page 287, are great with this! Store in the refrigerator for up to 3 days.

Photo on page 133.

Chicken Ranch Pitas

These pitas are so easy and so yummy that you'll find yourself making them all the time! I like to make a big batch of cooked chicken breast on Sundays so that I have precooked chicken ready and waiting for meals like this one, or you can just save your leftover chicken for this recipe. But whatever you do, don't buy precooked chicken. You want it to be fresh and free of chemicals and preservatives. Plus, it's so much cheaper to cook your own.

Makes 2 servings | Serving size: 1 pita | Per serving: calories 400; fat 22 g; saturated fat 8 g; fiber 7 g; protein 28 g; carbohydrates 25 g; sugar 2.5 g | Prep time: 5 minutes | Cook time: 0 minutes

2 small whole wheat pitas, cut in half
4 large romaine leaves
½ tomato, thinly sliced
4 thin red onion slices
1 cooked boneless, skinless chicken breast (see page 132)
1 avocado, thinly sliced
¼ cup shredded cheddar cheese
¼ cup Ranch Dip (page 160)

1. Carefully open each pita half to avoid tearing it. Add a romaine leaf to each pita half; if they don't fit, tear them and make them fit (you're the boss here!). Add a slice of tomato and onion to each pita half.

2. Slice the chicken breast and divide it among the 4 pita halves, top with avocado slices, sprinkle with the cheese, and drizzle some ranch dip over the top. If you're traveling with these, dress them just before eating.

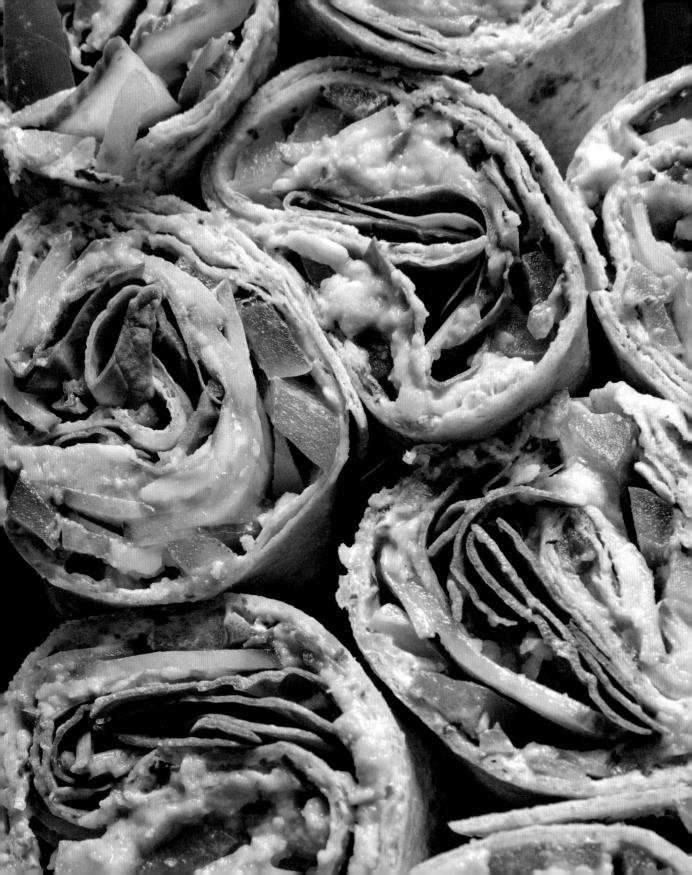

Veggie-Packed Pinwheels

These colorful little rounds of goodness will make you feel amazing; they're packed full of good-for-you ingredients and have tons of flavor, so you'll be hooked fast! They also make great appetizers for game day or after-school snacks for kiddos.

Makes 2 servings | Serving size: 4 pinwheels | Per serving: calories 442; fat 25 g; saturated fat 7 g; fiber 33 g; protein 13 g; carbohydrates 46 g; sugar 5 g | Prep time: 5 minutes | Cook time: 0 minutes

---

2 tablespoons cream cheese
2 tablespoons pesto (see page 107)
1 avocado
2 (10-inch) burrito-size whole wheat tortillas
1 red bell pepper, sliced into thin strips
½ cucumber, cut into thin slices
½ cup baby spinach

1. In a small bowl, stir together the cream cheese and pesto until smooth. In another small bowl, smash the avocado with the back of a fork.

2. Place the tortillas on a clean surface. Smear each with the pesto–cream cheese mixture, spreading it out to the edges.

3. Arrange the bell pepper and cucumber slices on top of the pesto–cream cheese mixture and dollop on the avocado, smearing it a little over the veggies (it doesn't have to be perfect; it's just to hold the veggies in the pinwheels). Top with spinach and roll up the wraps very tightly, like a sushi roll. Let them sit for 10 minutes to help them hold together (I like to clean up the kitchen while I wait).

4. Slice each wrap in half, then each half in half. These are big pinwheels. Enjoy!

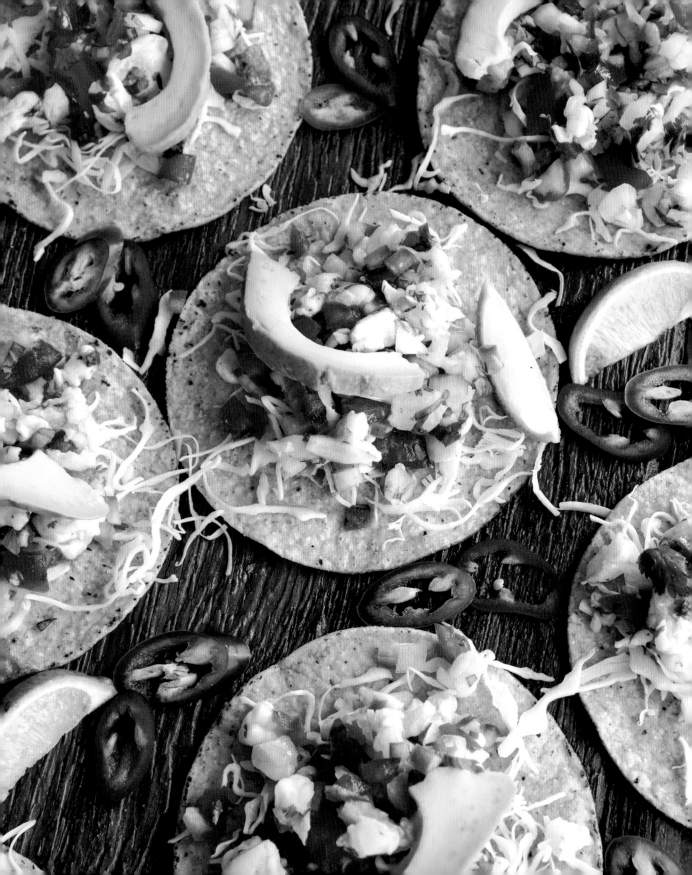

Ceviche Tostadas

I didn't even try to make my own recipe here; I just called my sister-in-law and asked for hers. So for the record, this is a Brenda Johns recipe, not an Audrey Johns recipe! Brenda makes the best ceviche I've ever had, and I was thrilled to work with her on this. We live about twenty-four hundred miles apart, but that didn't stop us! She messaged me her recipe, I tested it and asked some questions, and when I felt it was up to her high standards, I sent it back for approval. I know you'll love it, but if you don't, you can reach her at . . . Just kidding, haha.

You can find the tostadas next to tortillas in most grocery stores. If you can't find them, get yellow corn taco shells. Break the shells in half and you have a tostada (albeit cut in half), but these will do in a pinch.

One last tip: Get the freshest fish you can find. Ask your fishmonger for the freshest they have, or go to a fish market. Because you won't be applying any heat to the fish, you want the best possible quality.

Makes 6 servings | *Serving size: 2 tostadas* | *Per serving: calories 202; fat 6 g; saturated fat 2 g; fiber 2.5 g; protein 18 g; carbohydrates 19.5 g; sugar 4 g* | *Prep time: 20 minutes plus 2 hours marinating time*

1 pound tilapia or shrimp, peeled and deveined
Juice of 8 limes
6 plum tomatoes, chopped
2 serrano peppers, ribs and seeds removed, minced
2 jalapeños, ribs and seeds removed, minced
½ white onion, finely chopped
¼ cup chopped fresh cilantro
12 tostadas
1 avocado, sliced (optional)

1. Chop the fish or shrimp into ¼-inch cubes, adding it to a large nonreactive bowl as you work. Squeeze the lime juice on top, cover, and refrigerate for 2 hours to "cook" the fish in the lime juice. If you've never made fish this way, don't fret—the acid in the lime juice actually cures it and gives it a "cooked" consistency!

2. Meanwhile, place the tomatoes, serranos, jalapeños, onion, and cilantro in a medium bowl. Mix well and set aside, allowing the flavors to blend.

3. When the fish is done "cooking," pour off most of the juice, leaving about 2 tablespoons. Add the chopped veggies and mix well.

4. Top each tostada with about ¼ cup ceviche and a slice of avocado and enjoy.

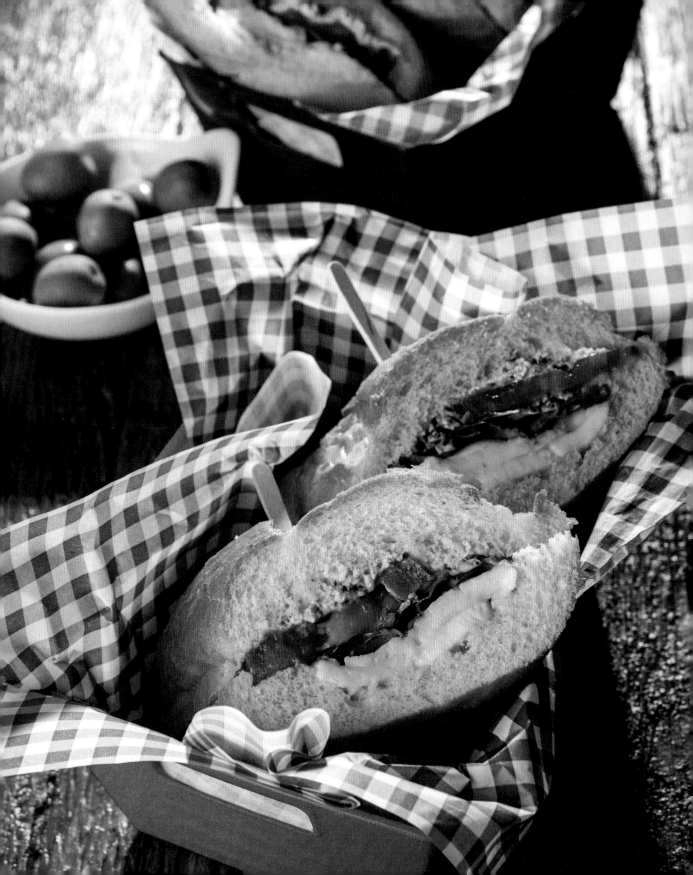

Caprice Pesto Sandwich

The first day I made this sandwich I sent a photo of it to my best friend, Kara. She'd just texted me a photo of her lunch, which consisted of grapes, cubed cheese, hummus, and pita chips, and she must have been jealous because she responded with texts like "You suck" and "I want *that*!" My yummy sandwich had far fewer calories than her lunch and was more exciting, too. I made it three more times that week and sent her photos every time.

I know what you're thinking—*This can't be healthy*! Well, I hollow out the rolls, removing all the bread I can, and use wholesome ingredients, including my skinny pesto (see page 107), for lots of flavor—and a deceptively healthy sandwich is born.

This is a vegetarian recipe; meat eaters can add shredded cooked chicken breast for added protein.

Makes 2 servings | Serving size: 1 sandwich | Per serving: calories 217; fat 12 g; saturated fat 4 g; fiber 2.5 g; protein 13 g; carbohydrates 16 g; sugar 5 g | Prep time: 10 minutes | Cook time: 0 minutes

---

2 hoagie rolls
2 medium tomatoes
2 tablespoons pesto (see page 107)
4 tablespoons 0% Greek yogurt
6 thin slices off an 8-ounce ball of mozzarella cheese, or 2 deli slices (you really should get the mozzarella ball—it's so much better here!)
20 fresh basil leaves

1. Cut the rolls in half and gently use your clean fingers to scoop out 80 percent of the soft inner bread, leaving just the crusts. Discard the inner bread or let it dry to make homemade bread crumbs.

2. In a small bowl, mix the pesto and yogurt. Smear the mixture on the top half of the rolls.

3. Place the cheese on the bottom halves of the rolls and top with the basil leaves, tomatoes, and the pesto-smeared tops. Halve and serve. If making them to go, roll up in paper towels to soak up any tomato juice and avoid soggy bread. Make sure you eat these the same day you make them, or the tomatoes will ruin the bread.

Lovely Lox Plate

We already know that smoked salmon is good for us, but who needs all that bread in a bagel? Okay, to be honest, I do, so I created this healthy plate to give myself the illusion of a big carbohydrate-packed meal.

If you have bagels in the house and want to use them in this recipe, just have half! Any other bread will work well, too—leftover sliced French bread is fantastic and so chic next to the salad and coral-colored fish. Go ahead and take a photo—you know you want to!

Makes 1 serving | Serving size: 1 plate | Per serving: calories 490; fat 20 g; saturated fat 2.5 g; fiber 5 g; protein 38.5 g; carbohydrates 40 g; sugar 13 g | Prep time: 10 minutes | Cook time: 0 minutes

1 slice whole wheat sourdough bread
3 ounces lox or smoked salmon (about 4 slices)
4 tomato slices
4 thin cucumber slices
1 teaspoon drained capers (optional)
Lemon wedge (optional)
1 tablespoon low-fat cream cheese
½ teaspoon chopped fresh dill
½ teaspoon chopped fresh chives
½ teaspoon extra-virgin olive oil
2 teaspoons balsamic vinegar
1 tablespoon fresh lemon juice
Pinch of kosher salt
Pinch of freshly ground black pepper
1 cup mixed baby greens
1 green onion, thinly sliced

1. Toast the bread, cut it in quarters, and place it on a large plate with the salmon and tomato and cucumber slices. Top the salmon with the capers and (if using) add the lemon wedge to the plate.

2. In a small bowl, mash together the cream cheese, dill, and chives and add to the plate next to the veggies.

3. In a large bowl, whisk together the oil, vinegar, lemon juice, salt, and pepper. Top with the greens and green onion and toss together. Add the salad to the plate with the salmon and enjoy.

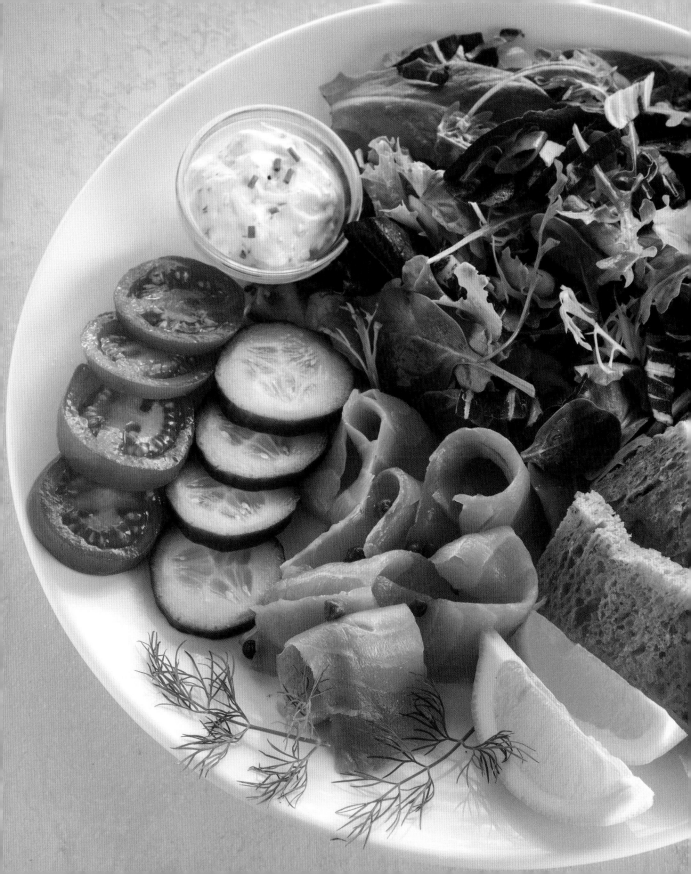

9

Make-Ahead Detox Meals

Slow cookers and freezer meals will save you on hectic weeks! And I'm not talking about those frozen dinners you get at the grocery store; I'm talking about a homemade tray of lasagna, French bread pizza, and chicken strips that require just a pop in the oven after a hard day of work.

A little meal planning and prep work on the weekend can save your sanity during the week. Knowing what you're having for dinner will stop you from mindlessly snacking on junk at the office or hitting the drive-thru on the way home.

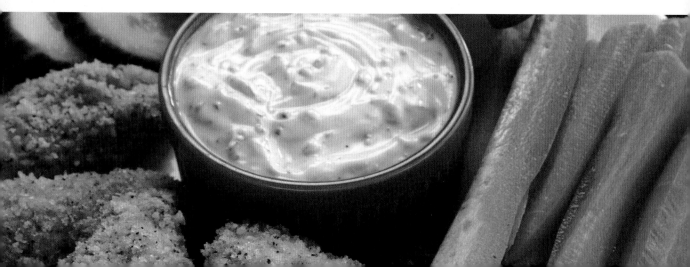

Slow Cooker "Chunky" Beef Stew

This stew is so easy and delicious that you won't believe how incredibly healthy it is! If you're looking to cut back on meat, or are vegetarian or vegan, you can easily make this a vegetable stew—simply skip the beef, replace the beef broth with vegetable broth, up the amount of vegetables, and top with cubed cooked tofu before serving (see page 134 for tofu cooking directions).

Now, I can already hear some of you saying, "Wine? I thought we were supposed to back off the booze!" Well, all the alcohol in the wine will cook off, and it adds an amazing flavor and complexity to the dish. And let's be honest here—if you're going to end up drinking a little glass of something while on these detox plans, red wine is the way to go. It's low in carbohydrates and high in potassium, magnesium, calcium, and iron, and it's actually good for your heart, but if you still want to skip the booze (good for you, love), just replace the wine with more beef broth.

Makes 10 servings | *Serving size: 1 cup* | *Per serving: calories 205; fat 8 g; saturated fat 3 g; fiber 2 g; protein 13 g; carbohydrates 15.5 g; sugar 2.5 g* | *Prep time: 20 minutes* | *Cook time: 3 to 6 hours (in a slow cooker)*

1 tablespoon olive oil
1¼ pounds lean beef stew meat, cut into 1-inch cubes
2 tablespoons all-purpose flour
1 teaspoon paprika
2 garlic cloves, chopped
1 medium yellow onion, chopped
1 pound Yukon Gold potatoes, cut into 1-inch dice
4 small carrots, cut into 1-inch chunks
8 ounces white mushrooms, halved
4 celery stalks, cut into 1-inch chunks
3 cups beef broth or bone broth
2 tablespoons tomato paste
1 teaspoon chopped fresh rosemary
4 fresh sage leaves, chopped
1 cup dry red wine or more beef broth

1. In a large skillet, heat the oil over medium-high heat.

2. In a deep bowl or gallon-size freezer bag, combine the beef, flour, and paprika and toss until all the beef is coated. Add the beef to the skillet in a single layer, taking care not to crowd it (if your skillet is too small, work in batches). Cook for 2 to 3 minutes on each side, just until the beef browns a little. Transfer the beef to a slow cooker.

3. Top the browned meat with the garlic, onion, potatoes, carrots, mushrooms, and celery.

4. In the bowl or bag you used for the stew meat, combine 1 cup of the broth, the tomato paste, rosemary, and sage. Mix until smooth, then add the mixture to the slow cooker along with the remaining 2 cups broth and the wine.

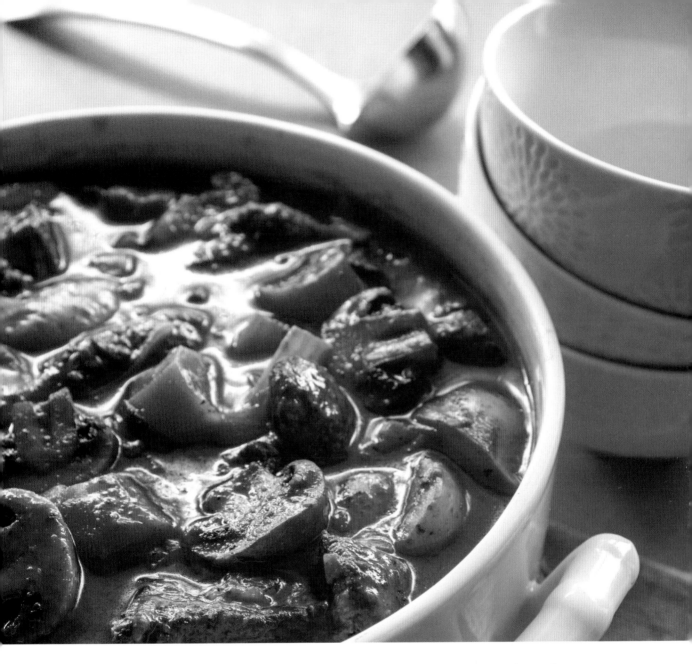

5. Cover the slow cooker and cook on high for 3 hours or on low for 6 to 9 hours (the longer you cook it, the better it is!).

6. I like to uncover the slow cooker for the last hour to help thicken up the sauce, so

if you like a thicker sauce, go for it. If you prefer a thinner, more soup-like consistency, just leave it alone. Serve hot. Store leftover stew in an airtight container in the refrigerator for up to 3 days or in the freezer for up to 3 months.

Chicken, Rice, and Black Bean Burrito Bowl

This meal may take a little extra effort, but if you make enough, you'll have lunches ready to go for a whole week. And let's be honest, it's only a little more work because you need a pot and sauté pan going at the same time, which, to me, is high-maintenance cooking. . . .

I like to double this recipe. I make it for dinner, and then after we've eaten, I pack up the leftovers into individual containers for lunches. My family *loves* these burrito bowls, so I might as well get dinner and a week's worth of lunches done all at once, right?

Makes 5 servings | *Serving size: ⅓ cup rice and beans, ½ cup chicken and veggies, and 1 tablespoon cheese* | *Per serving: calories 160; fat 3 g; saturated fat 1 g; fiber 6.5 g; protein 18 g; carbohydrates 45 g; sugar 5 g* | *Prep time: 15 minutes* | *Cook time: 30 minutes*

¾ cup uncooked brown rice
1½ cups vegetable broth
1 teaspoon olive oil
1 red bell pepper, chopped into ¼-inch cubes
1 medium red onion, chopped into ¼-inch cubes
1 jalapeño, ribs and seeds removed, minced
Pinch of kosher salt
2 boneless, skinless chicken breasts, cut into ½-inch cubes
2 tomatoes, chopped into ¼-inch dice
3 garlic cloves, chopped
¼ cup frozen corn, thawed
¼ cup chopped fresh cilantro
1 green onion, thinly sliced
1 (15-ounce) can black beans, drained and rinsed (preferably BPA-free cans)

OPTIONAL TOPPINGS
Grated sharp cheddar cheese
Chopped fresh cilantro
Hot sauce or salsa
Diced avocado
0% Greek yogurt
Lime wedges

1. In a small saucepan, stir together the rice and broth. Cover and bring to a low boil over medium heat, then turn the heat to low and cook, undisturbed, until all the liquid is absorbed, 15 to 20 minutes.

2. Meanwhile, heat the oil in a large sauté pan over medium heat. Add the bell pepper, onion, jalapeño, and salt and sauté until the vegetables are soft, about 10 minutes. Add the chicken, tomatoes, garlic, and corn and sauté for about 15 minutes, until the chicken is cooked through, with no pink in the cubes.

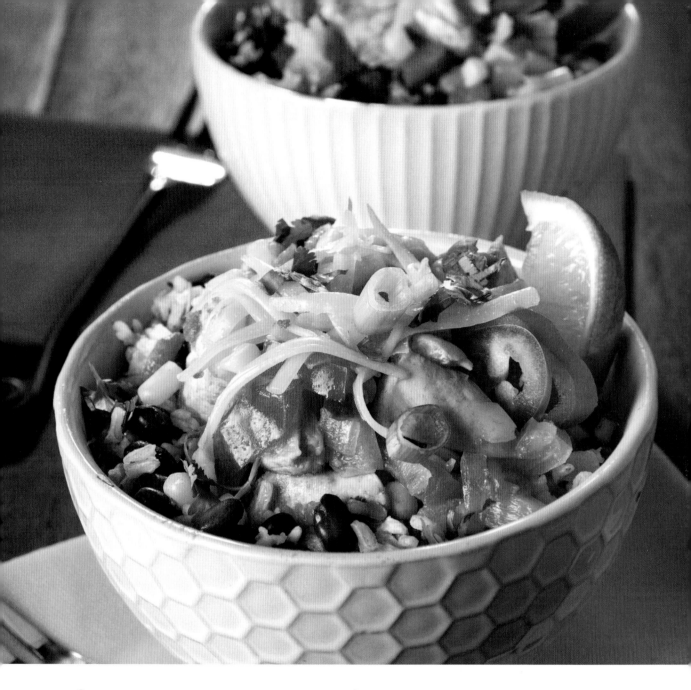

3. Stir the cilantro, green onion, and beans into the cooked rice, cover, and set aside to heat the beans in the rice.

4. To plate, place ⅓ cup of the rice and beans in a bowl (or travel container) and top with ½ cup of the chicken and veggies. I like to top mine with cheese, yogurt, and my favorite hot sauce, but choose your own toppings. Store leftovers in an airtight container in the refrigerator for up to 3 days.

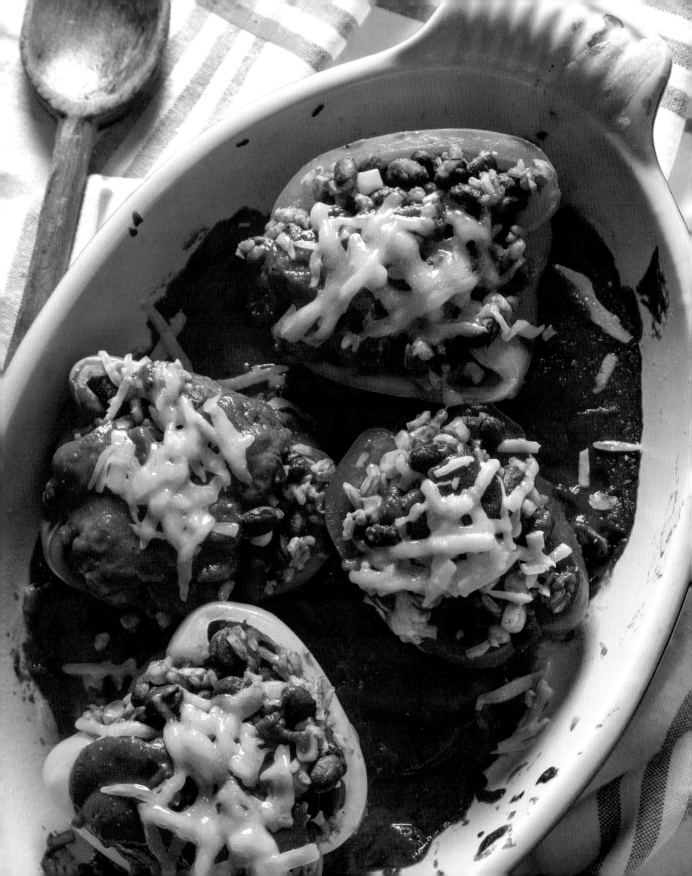

Stuffed Bell Pepper Casserole

Stuffed bell peppers are actually very easy to make, but many people are put off by all the stuffing "work," so I took the stress out of it and created a casserole version. All you do is halve the peppers, dump the filling over all of them (spillage between the peppers is both fine and encouraged), and bake. No worrying that they will fall over and lose all their filling in the oven, and they're easier to serve and dig into than whole peppers.

Have a favorite stuffed bell pepper recipe? Try this method—easy-peasy, yummy, and cheesy!

Makes 4 servings | Serving size: 1 bell pepper half | Per serving: calories 288; fat 5 g; saturated fat 2 g; fiber 10 g; protein 11.5 g; carbohydrates 48 g; sugar 8 g | Prep time: 20 minutes | Cook time: 45 minutes

½ cup uncooked brown rice
1¼ cups vegetable, chicken, beef, or bone broth
Olive oil spray
2 bell peppers, any color
1 (15-ounce) can black beans (preferably BPA-free cans)
1 (6-ounce) can tomato paste (preferably BPA-free can)
1 teaspoon garlic powder
¼ teaspoon chili powder
⅛ teaspoon freshly ground black pepper
Dash of hot sauce (optional)
¼ cup frozen corn, thawed
¼ cup shredded sharp cheddar cheese

1. In a small saucepan, stir together the rice and broth. Cover and bring to a low boil over medium heat, then turn the heat to low and cook, undisturbed, until all the liquid is absorbed, 15 to 20 minutes.

2. Preheat the oven to 350°F. Spray a 9 × 9-inch casserole dish with oil spray.

3. Halve the bell peppers from top to bottom, remove the seeds, ribs, and stems, and place the pepper halves cut side up in the casserole dish.

4. Drain the liquid from the beans into a medium bowl and add ⅓ cup water, the tomato paste, garlic powder, chili powder, black pepper, and hot sauce (if using). Set aside.

5. In a large bowl, combine the cooked rice, beans, corn, and tomato paste mixture. Divide this filling among the prepared bell pepper halves. If some spills out between the peppers, that's okay.

6. Top with the cheese and bake for 35 to 45 minutes, until the cheese is melted and the peppers are soft. Each serving is 1 bell pepper half. Store leftover casserole in the refrigerator for up to 3 days or in the freezer for up to 3 months.

Vegetarian Lasagna

You won't even miss the meat in this hearty lasagna! I added three veggies that all mimic meat, plus with all the cheese and sauce your taste buds (and your family) will be too distracted to even notice they're eating healthy! If you absolutely must have meat in your lasagna, I've given some options in the variations below.

This lasagna freezes beautifully; I always make two trays and freeze one for fast weeknight meals.

Makes 4 servings | *Serving size: 1 slice (about 1½ cups)* | *Per serving: calories 360; fat 13 g; saturated fat 6.5 g; fiber 12 g; protein 16 g; carbohydrates 49 g; sugar 13 g*
Prep time: 60 minutes | *Cook time: 50 minutes plus 20 minutes rest time*

1 cup ⅛-inch-diced eggplant
1 tablespoon kosher salt
1 cup ⅛-inch-diced zucchini
1 cup diced white mushrooms
¼ cup mascarpone cheese, at room temperature
2 tablespoons chopped fresh basil
⅔ cup shredded mozzarella cheese
3 cups marinara sauce (see page 155)
6 no-bake lasagna sheets

1. Cover a baking sheet with two layers of paper towels. Spread the eggplant on top, sprinkle with the salt, and toss. Cover the eggplant with two more layers of paper towels and leave for 1 hour on the countertop or in the fridge all day. This will help draw out some moisture and give the eggplant a meatier texture.

2. Place the eggplant, zucchini, mushrooms, mascarpone, and basil in a large bowl and toss everything together.

3. Spread ⅓ cup marinara sauce in the bottom of a 9 × 9-inch casserole dish. Layer as follows: 2 lasagna sheets, half the veggie mixture, 2 lasagna sheets, ⅓ cup sauce, the remaining veggies, 2 lasagna sheets, and the rest of the sauce. Cover with foil and let sit for 20 minutes so that the sauce can soak into the pasta.

4. Preheat the oven to 375°F.

5. Bake the lasagna, covered, for 30 minutes, then uncover and sprinkle the mozzarella on top. Bake for 20 minutes, or until the cheese is melted and the sauce is bubbling. Let it rest for 20 minutes; this will help keep the lasagna together when you cut into it. Divide among four plates and serve. Store leftover lasagna in an airtight container in the refrigerator for up to 3 days or in the freezer for up to 3 months.

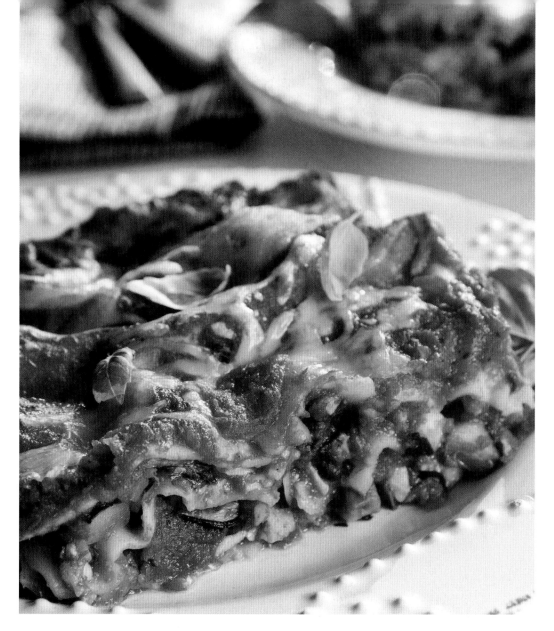

VARIATIONS

- In a skillet over medium heat, thoroughly cook a turkey or chicken Italian sausage. Cut it in half lengthwise and remove the meat from the casing. Discard the casing and crumble the meat into the bowl with the veggies.

- In a skillet over medium heat, brown ¼ pound ground turkey, crumbling it as you cook. Add 1 teaspoon Italian seasoning, 1 teaspoon grated Parmesan, and a pinch each of salt and pepper. Drain the meat of any liquid and mix in 2 tablespoons of the marinara sauce. Add the meat to the veggies.

- If you like things spicy, mix ½ to 1 tablespoon red pepper flakes with the marinara sauce.

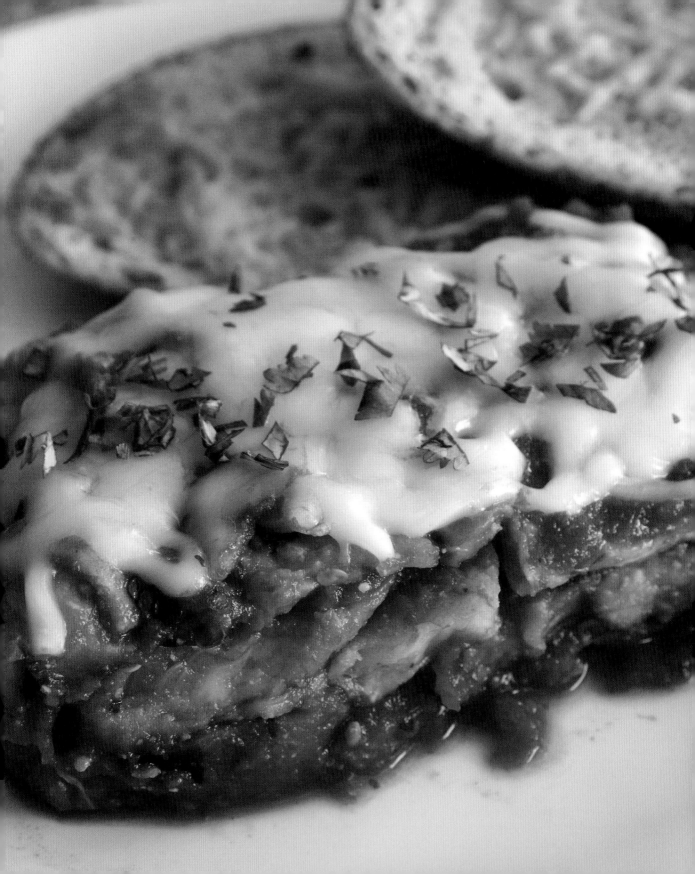

Eggplant Parmesan and Garlic Toast

This is my go-to Meatless Monday dish; I like to get it started in the morning and then assemble it when I get home, but you can also prep everything and put it in the fridge so you don't have to bother with the assembly after being on your feet all day. You choose! Here are my tips to an easy make-ahead meal:

1. Use your slow cooker! I like to make the sauce in the slow cooker so I can walk away and forget about it for hours.
2. Make it in the a.m.! I start the slow cooker in the morning and "sweat" the eggplant in the fridge while I'm working. It takes me about 10 minutes of prep, and I can walk away for the rest of the day.
3. Get it done on your day off! You can completely assemble this dish and place in the fridge or freezer—just pop it in the oven when you get home and kick off your shoes.

Makes 4 servings | Serving size: 1½ cups eggplant Parmesan and 1 slice of garlic toast
Per serving: calories 411; fat 10.5 g; saturated fat 4 g; fiber 18.5 g; protein 17.5 g; carbohydrates 44 g; sugar 22 g | Prep time: 2 hours (most of this is the eggplants sweating) | Cook time: 5 hours (most of this can be done in a slow cooker)

MARINARA SAUCE

1 teaspoon olive oil
1 medium yellow or white onion, finely chopped
Kosher salt
4 garlic cloves, chopped
1 (28-ounce) can crushed tomatoes (look for BPA-free cans)
1 (15-ounce) can tomato sauce
1 (6-ounce) can tomato paste
Pinch of freshly ground black pepper
Pinch of raw organic sugar (it cuts the acid in the tomatoes—and, babe, it's just a pinch!)
3 tablespoons chopped fresh basil, or 1 tablespoon Italian seasoning

EGGPLANT PARMESAN

1 large eggplant (about 2 pounds)
3 teaspoons kosher salt
Olive oil spray
½ cup shredded mozzarella cheese
3 teaspoons freshly grated Parmesan cheese

GARLIC TOAST

4 slices good whole wheat sourdough or French bread
1⅓ tablespoons butter (I love Earth Balance vegan butter, but you can use any butter here)
4 teaspoons freshly grated Parmesan cheese
2 teaspoons garlic powder
1 tablespoon chopped fresh basil (optional)

(recipe continues)

1. Make the marinara sauce: Heat the oil in a large saucepan over medium heat. Add the onion and a pinch of salt and sauté for about 5 minutes, until soft. Add the garlic and cook for 5 minutes, or until the onion is mostly transparent. (If using a slow cooker, you can use a skillet instead of a large saucepan. Once cooked, transfer the onion and garlic to the slow cooker after the onion is transparent and turn the heat on low.)

2. Add the crushed tomatoes, tomato sauce, tomato paste, pepper, sugar, and basil and mix to combine. Bring to a boil, then cover, reduce the heat to low, and simmer for 4 hours, stirring every hour to avoid burning. (In a slow cooker, cook on low for 5 to 8 hours or on high for 3 to 4 hours.)

3. Make the eggplant Parmesan: Line a rimmed baking sheet with two layers of paper towels and sprinkle with ¾ teaspoon of the salt. Peel the eggplant, using a vegetable peeler or knife. Cut the eggplant into ½-inch-thick rounds and lay them in a single layer on the baking sheet. Sprinkle with ¾ teaspoon of the salt, top with two more layers of paper towels, sprinkle with ¾ teaspoon of the salt, add a second layer of eggplant, sprinkle with the remaining ¾ teaspoon salt, and top with two layers of paper towels. This will sweat out most of the moisture and ensure that your meal is not a soupy mess.

4. Let the eggplant sit for 2 to 10 hours in the fridge, then remove the paper towels. Line two baking sheets with parchment paper and spread the eggplant rounds in an even layer on the prepared baking sheets. Spray lightly with oil spray, flip, and spray lightly with oil spray again.

5. Preheat the oven to 350°F.

6. Bake the eggplant for 10 minutes, flip, and bake for about 10 minutes more, until soft. Set aside.

7. Spread ⅓ cup of marinara sauce in the bottom of a 9 × 13-inch baking dish. Layer as follows: a single layer of eggplant, ⅓ cup sauce, 1½ teaspoons Parmesan, the rest of the eggplant, 1½ cups sauce, the remaining Parmesan, and the mozzarella. If you are making this ahead, cover and move to the fridge or freezer now (just be sure to thaw completely before baking).

8. Bake for 35 minutes, uncovered, or until the cheese is melted and slightly browned. Let it sit for 15 minutes to help it hold together for serving.

9. Meanwhile, make the garlic toast: Place the bread slices on a baking sheet, spread the tops with the butter, and sprinkle with the Parmesan and garlic powder. Bake for 10 minutes, or until the cheese starts to brown, then cut each slice in half and sprinkle with the basil (if using).

10. Divide the eggplant Parmesan among four large plates and serve it with the garlic toast. Store leftovers in an airtight container in the refrigerator for up to 3 days or in the freezer for up to 3 months.

Chicken Soup in a Slow Cooker

This easy slow cooker meal is perfect for hectic schedules—just toss everything in, turn it on, and head to work. Make it in the morning and come home to a delicious dinner and a house that smells amazing!

Makes 5 servings | *Serving size: 2 cups* | *Per serving: calories 141; fat 1 g; saturated fat 0 g; fiber 3.5 g; protein 17.6 g; carbohydrates 16 g; sugar 6 g* | *Prep time: 20 minutes* | *Cook time: 8 hours (in a slow cooker)*

2 boneless, skinless chicken breasts
2 parsnips, peeled and chopped into ¼-inch cubes
2 carrots, chopped into ¼-inch cubes
1 medium yellow onion, chopped
2 celery stalks, chopped into ¼-inch cubes
2 teaspoons garlic powder
2 teaspoons kosher salt
½ teaspoon freshly ground black pepper
2 bay leaves
7 cups (1¾ quarts) chicken broth
Juice of ½ lemon
3 tablespoons chopped fresh flat-leaf parsley

1. Place the chicken, parsnips, carrots, onion, celery, garlic powder, salt, pepper, bay leaves, and broth in a slow cooker. Turn the slow cooker to high, cover, and cook for 8 hours.

2. Carefully remove the chicken breasts and shred with two forks. Add the shredded chicken back to the soup and cook for another 10 minutes.

3. When you're ready to serve, stir in the lemon juice. Taste for seasoning and add more salt and pepper as needed. Ladle into bowls, top with the parsley, and serve. Store leftover soup in an airtight container in the refrigerator for up to 3 days or in the freezer for up to 3 months.

Photo on page 57.

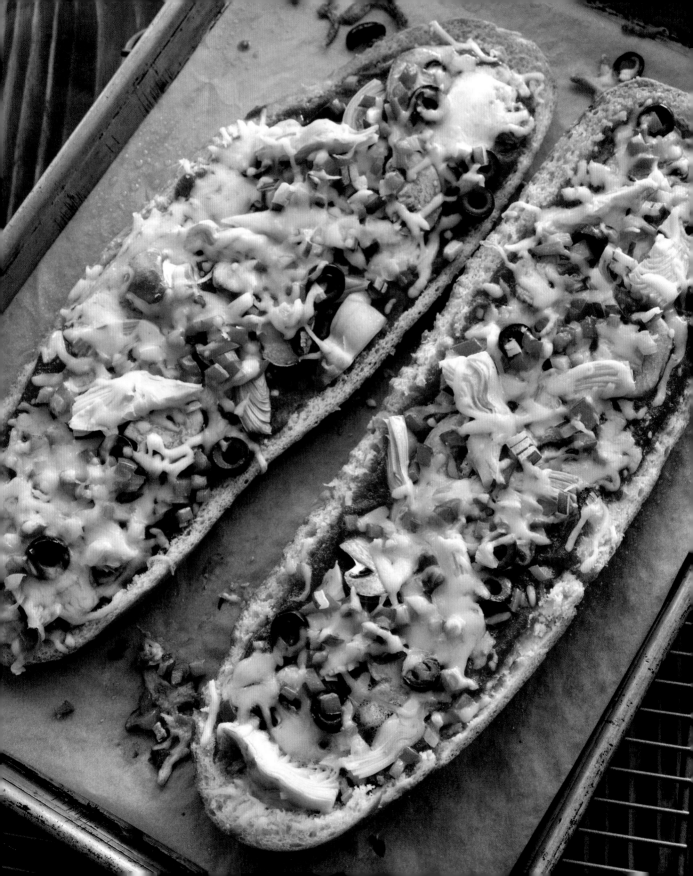

Vegetarian French Bread Pizza

I know what you're thinking: *How on earth can I eat French bread pizza and lose weight?* Well, I really do a number on the poor loaf of bread—I take out almost all the inside of the bread, saving calories and unnecessary carbohydrates.

So try this baby out, and don't feel bad if you let out an evil laugh while destroying the loaf of bread—I always do!

Makes 4 servings | *Serving size: ½ French bread pizza* | *Per serving: calories 232; fat 8 g; saturated fat 5 g; fiber 4 g; protein 11 g; carbohydrates 29 g; sugar 7 g* | *Prep time: 15 minutes* | *Cook time: 20 minutes*

---

1 (8-ounce) can tomato sauce
2 tablespoons tomato paste
10 large fresh basil leaves, chopped
2 garlic cloves, chopped
Kosher salt and freshly ground black pepper
1 large French baguette
1 cup shredded mozzarella cheese
2 red or green bell peppers, cut into ⅛-inch dice
¼ cup diced red onion
1 cup sliced white mushrooms
3 tablespoons sliced canned black olives
3 canned artichoke hearts, roughly chopped

1. In a medium bowl, mix together the tomato sauce, tomato paste, basil, garlic, and a pinch each of salt and black pepper. Set aside to marinate for at least 1 hour, but you can do this up to 24 hours ahead of time.

2. Preheat the oven to 375°F.

3. Slice the bread lengthwise in thirds. Reserve the middle third to make bread crumbs, French toast, or croutons (see page 79).

4. Hollow out the top and bottom halves of the bread, leaving a layer of bread ¼ inch thick all the way around.

5. Place the tops and bottoms of the bread cut side up on a rimmed baking sheet. Spread half the pizza sauce over each piece of bread and top with the cheese, bell peppers, onion, mushrooms, olives, and artichoke hearts.

6. Bake for 15 to 20 minutes, until the cheese has melted and the bread is golden and crispy along the edges.

7. Let the pizzas cool for 5 minutes, then cut each pizza into 8 slices and serve (a single serving is 4 slices). Store leftovers in an airtight container in the refrigerator for up to 3 days or in the freezer for up to 3 months.

Crunchy Cheddar Chicken Strips with Ranch Dip and Veggie Sticks

For the kid in all of us, an entire meal that consists of finger foods! The chicken strips can be made ahead and frozen for fast weeknight meals; you can also prep them in the morning and bake them when you get home from work. You'll be eating in ten minutes!

The ranch dip can be made 2 or 3 days ahead of time, and you can even chop the veggies when you bring them home from grocery shopping and store them in airtight containers.

Makes 4 servings | *Serving size: 3 chicken strips, ¼ cup ranch dip, and as many veggies as you want* | *Per serving: calories 443; fat 6.5 g; saturated fat 2.5 g; fiber 2.5 g; protein 65 g; carbohydrates 28 g; sugar 7 g* | *Prep time: 15 minutes* | *Cook time: 20 minutes*

1 cup panko bread crumbs
3 tablespoons finely shredded sharp cheddar cheese
1 teaspoon chili powder
½ teaspoon kosher salt
¼ teaspoon freshly ground black pepper
1 egg
2 pounds chicken tenderloins

RANCH DIP AND VEGGIES
1 cup 0% Greek yogurt
1 garlic clove
1 tablespoon minced fresh chives
1 tablespoon minced fresh flat-leaf parsley
1 tablespoon minced fresh dill
1 teaspoon white vinegar
Kosher salt and freshly ground black pepper
1 red bell pepper, cut into thin strips
1 cucumber, sliced into ¼-inch-thick rounds
4 carrots, cut into ¼-inch-thick sticks

1. Preheat the oven to 350°F. Line two baking sheets with parchment paper.

2. In a pie pan or large shallow bowl, mix together the bread crumbs, cheese, chili powder, salt, and pepper until the cheese is evenly distributed; if it sticks together, roll the mixture in the palms of your hands and it will break it up.

3. In another pie pan, whisk the egg. Dip each chicken tenderloin in the egg, then thoroughly coat with the bread crumbs. Lay them on the prepared baking sheets as you finish.

4. Bake the chicken strips for 20 minutes, or until golden and cooked through (no pink on the inside and juices run clear).

5. Meanwhile, make the ranch dip: Place the yogurt in a medium bowl. Use a fine grater or garlic press to shred the garlic clove into the yogurt. If using a grater, grate just about two-thirds of the clove, so you don't cut yourself, and discard the rest. If using a garlic press, just discard whatever is left in the press.

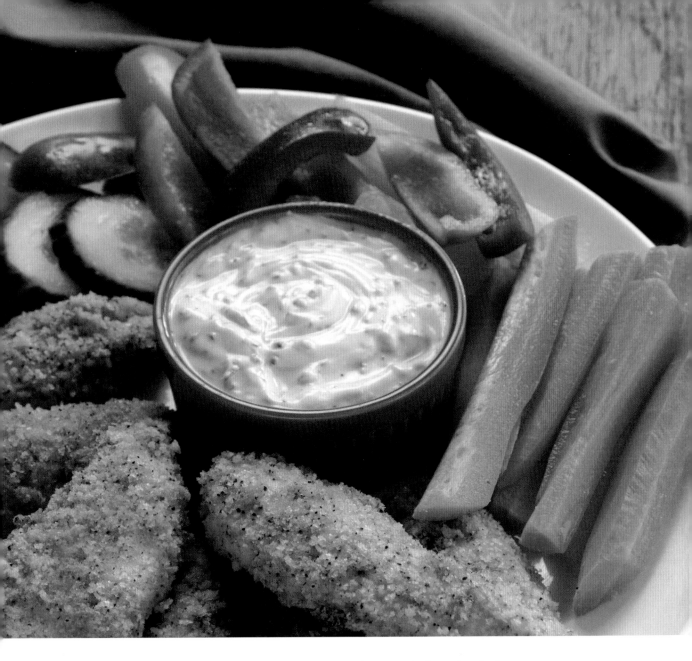

6. Add the chives, parsley, dill, vinegar, and salt and pepper to taste. Mix well and set aside until you're ready to serve.

7. To serve, divide the veggie sticks among four plates and place 3 chicken strips on each plate. Serve each plate with ¼ cup of the ranch dip. The chicken strips are amazing in the dip; it's not just for the veggies! Store leftover chicken strips in airtight containers in the refrigerator for up to 3 days or in the freezer for up to 3 months.

10

30-Minute Detox Meals

I wanted to share some of my favorite fast meals in this book! All of these can be made in just 30 minutes or less and are completely divine. These are great meals for new cooks; none are too daunting or difficult for first timers, and my seven-year-old daughter can make many of them (not kidding!), so be brave and dive in. Kitchen confidence is sexy!!

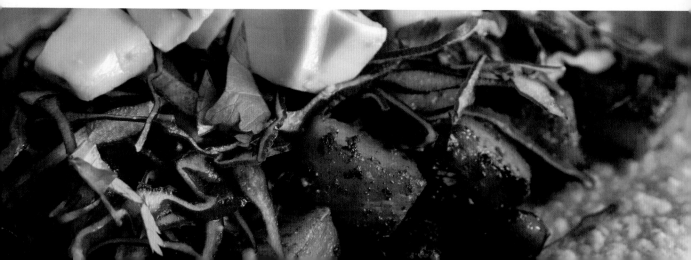

Surf-and-Turf Fajitas

A childhood friend, Ted, became a brilliant chef, and wouldn't you know it, he ended up as the head chef at the Texas restaurant known for creating the demand for fajitas! So when it came time to test this recipe I sent it off to Ted to test and receive his stamp of approval. You'll be pleased to know that this is not only a healthy dish, but it also comes with the Super Fajita Chef stamp of approval . . . which isn't really a thing, but it should be, don't you think?

If you don't like shrimp, use chicken breast—just slice it into thin strips, add it to the marinade with the steak, and cook for an additional 3 minutes. It's just that easy.

Makes 8 servings | Serving size: ½ cup fajita mixture and 1 tortilla | Per serving: calories 373; fat 15 g; saturated fat 5 g; fiber 4 g; protein 31.5 g; carbohydrates 28 g; sugar 5 g
Prep time: 10 minutes | Cook time: 15 minutes

Juice of 2 limes
1 teaspoon garlic powder
1 teaspoon ground cumin
1 teaspoon chili powder
½ teaspoon cayenne
1 teaspoon Italian seasoning
1 (1-pound) sirloin steak, sliced into thin strips against the grain
2 teaspoons olive oil
1 green bell pepper, cut into thin strips
1 red bell pepper, cut into thin strips
1 yellow bell pepper, cut into thin strips
1 medium yellow onion, cut into thin rings
1 jalapeño, ribs and seeds removed, cut into thin strips (optional)
Pinch of kosher salt
1 pound extra-large shrimp, peeled and deveined
8 (8-inch) whole wheat tortillas

OPTIONAL TOPPINGS
Salsa
0% Greek yogurt
Fresh or pickled jalapeño slices
Guacamole
Lime wedges

1. In a gallon-size freezer bag, combine the lime juice, garlic powder, cumin, chili powder, cayenne, Italian seasoning, and steak. Seal the bag and shake and squish until the meat is well coated in the marinade. Marinate for at least 30 minutes and up to 3 hours in the fridge.

2. In a large skillet, heat the oil over medium heat. Add the bell peppers, onion, jalapeño (if using), and salt and sauté until the bell peppers and onion start to soften, about 10 minutes. Transfer the vegetables to a plate, but leave the skillet on the heat.

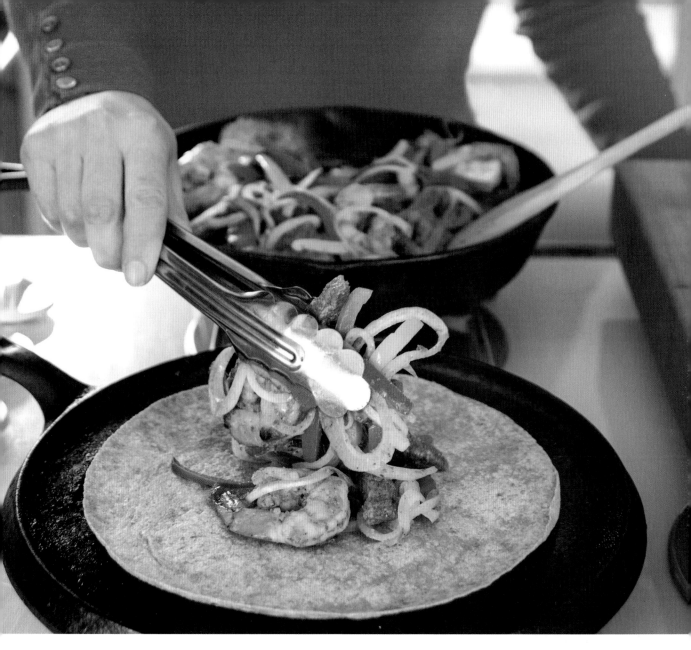

3. Remove the steak from the marinade and add to the skillet. Transfer the shrimp to the marinade (don't do this earlier, or the lime juice will "cook" the shrimp) while the steak cooks.

4. Cook the steak for 3 minutes, flipping to brown on all sides, then add the shrimp and marinade to the skillet. Toss together and cook for 2 minutes. Return the vegetables to the skillet and cook for 1 minute to heat them through.

5. Serve with the tortillas and toppings of your choice.

Pineapple Fried Rice

Disclaimer: You'll fight over the leftovers! I kid you not—I hoard them in the back of the fridge and write notes on it, like "You eat and you die." I'm not proud of this, but it's the truth, so if you make this and get into a big fight over the leftovers, you have been warned!

For those of you who have never heard of pineapple fried rice, no, it's not a Chinese dish but a Thai dish, and my favorite one, too! The pineapple gives a great sweet bite, and when you pair it with the crunchy cashews, you'll be in heaven.

Makes 4 servings | *Serving size: about 1 cup* | *Per serving: calories 463; fat 18 g; saturated fat 3.5 g; fiber 6.5 g; protein 20.5 g; carbohydrates 59 g; sugar 13 g* | *Prep time: 10 minutes* | *Cook time: 15 minutes*

²/₃ cup uncooked brown rice
2 large eggs
Olive oil spray
2 cups frozen or fresh pineapple chunks
1 boneless, skinless chicken breast, cut into thin strips
2 red bell peppers, cut into ½-inch dice
5 green onions, sliced on the diagonal
2 garlic cloves, minced
½ cup whole cashews
1 tablespoon reduced-sodium soy sauce
1 teaspoon sriracha, plus more to taste (optional)
Juice of ½ lime
¼ cup roughly chopped cilantro

1. In a small saucepan, stir together the rice and 1⅓ cups water. Cover and bring to a low boil over medium heat, then turn the heat to low and cook, undisturbed, until all the liquid is absorbed, 15 to 20 minutes.

2. Refrigerate the cooked rice for at least 15 minutes or preferably overnight (I make it the night before).

3. In a medium bowl, whisk the eggs.

4. Spray a wok or large skillet with oil spray and place over high heat. Add the eggs to the skillet and cook for about 1 minute, until they just start to set. Transfer the eggs back to the bowl you whisked them in.

5. Spray the skillet with more oil and add the pineapple, chicken, and bell peppers. Cook over high heat for 5 minutes, then lower the heat to medium, add the green onions and garlic, and cook for 2 minutes. Transfer everything to the bowl with the cooked eggs.

6. Add the cashews and the cold rice to the pan and sauté for 3 minutes. Return the contents of the bowl to the skillet, add the soy sauce, sriracha (if using), and lime juice, and cook for another 5 minutes over medium heat.

7. Top with the cilantro and more sriracha (if you like it spicy) . . . and don't forget to hide the leftovers in the back of the fridge so you won't have to share them!

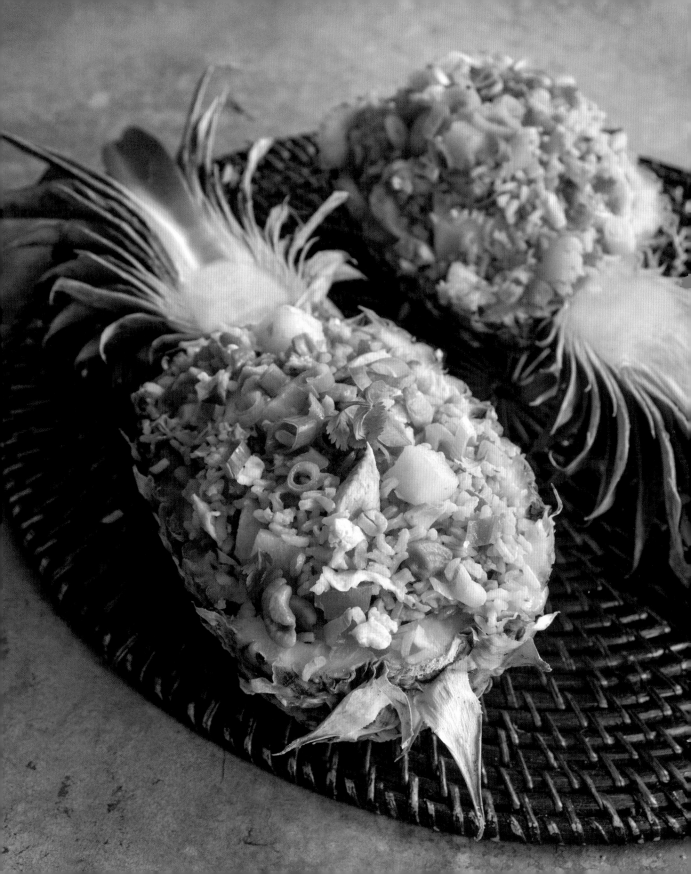

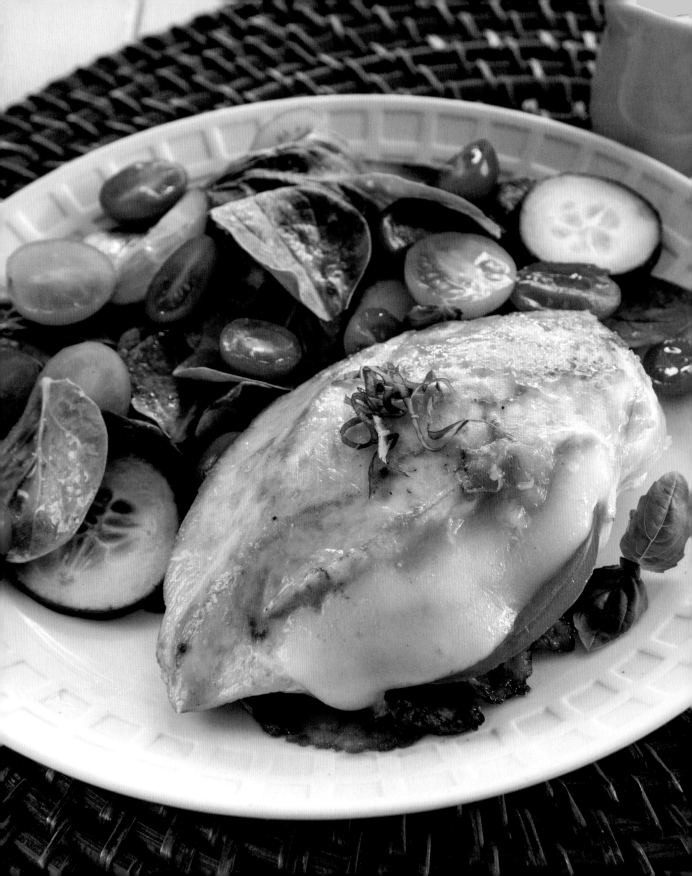

Caprese-Stuffed Chicken over a Simple Spinach Salad

I love this easy, delicious, and impressive 30-minute meal! To make it even faster, stuff the chicken breasts the morning or the night before, and throw them in the fridge. Then when you get home from work all you have to do is toss them in the pan and kick off your shoes.

Makes 4 servings | Serving size: 1 chicken breast and about ½ cup salad
Per serving: calories 280; fat 13 g; saturated fat 5 g; fiber 1 g; protein 35 g;
carbohydrates 5 g; sugar 2.5 g | Prep time: 10 minutes | Cook time: 25 minutes

CHICKEN
2 teaspoons olive oil
4 boneless, skinless chicken breasts
1 large tomato, cut into 8 slices
4 (⅛-inch-thick) mozzarella slices
⅛ teaspoon kosher salt
10 to 12 fresh basil leaves, thinly sliced

SALAD
2 teaspoons balsamic vinegar
1 teaspoon extra-virgin olive oil (basil olive oil is great here if you have it)
1 tablespoon freshly squeezed orange juice
2 cups baby spinach
4 (1-inch) pieces cucumber, sliced into thin rings
1 large tomato, cut into ½-inch cubes

1. Make the chicken: Heat the oil in a large sauté pan over medium heat.

2. Cut the chicken breasts in half horizontally by placing the palm of your hand on the top of a breast and using a sharp small knife to carefully cut it open like a pita, leaving one side intact and the other side open.

3. Place 2 tomato slices inside of each chicken breast, pushing them out to the sides so they don't overlap much, if at all. Place a slice of mozzarella on top of the tomatoes. Sprinkle the chicken breasts with the salt.

4. Gently place the chicken breasts in the hot sauté pan and let them cook undisturbed for 12 minutes, then flip and cook the other side for 10 to 12 minutes, until cooked through (no pink on the inside and the juices run clear). Some cheese will spill out as the breasts cook, and that's fine—the crunchy cheese is the best part!

5. Make the salad: While the chicken is cooking, pour the vinegar, oil, and orange juice into a small bowl or mason jar with a tight-fitting lid and whisk or shake vigorously to combine.

6. To serve, on each plate place ½ cup spinach and top with cucumber slices and tomato cubes. Place a chicken breast next to it, give the dressing a whisk, and drizzle it over the salad and chicken. Sprinkle the chicken with the sliced basil and serve.

Chicken and Avocado Grilled Cheese with Soup du Jour

I love this sandwich, and I make it often for last-minute dinners and weekend lunches on cold days. There's truly nothing better than dunking a fancy grilled cheese into a yummy homemade soup. Which soup, you ask? This sandwich goes great with both Tomato Basil Soup and Pesto Pea Soup. I like to freeze leftover soup just for this reason—for fast weeknight meals that taste like they took all day to make!

Makes 4 servings | Serving size: 1 sandwich and 1 cup soup | Per serving (just the sandwich; see pages 56 and 58 for soup nutrition): calories 478; fat 17 g; saturated fat 7 g; fiber 10 g; protein 28.5 g; carbohydrates 53 g; sugar 0 g | Prep time: 10 minutes | Cook time: 15 minutes

1 avocado
8 slices whole wheat sourdough bread
1 cup shredded sharp cheddar cheese
1 cup cooked, shredded chicken
Olive oil spray
4 cups Tomato Basil Soup (page 56) or Pesto Pea Soup (page 58)

1. In a small bowl, mash the avocado with the back of a fork.

2. Place 4 slices of the bread on a clean surface and sprinkle each slice with 2 tablespoons of the cheese. Arrange the shredded chicken over the cheese and top with the mashed avocado, the remaining cheese, and a slice of bread.

3. Lightly spray a large sauté pan with oil spray and place the sandwiches on the oiled surface. Lightly spray the tops with more oil.

4. Cover the sauté pan and heat over medium-low heat for 5 to 8 minutes per side, until the bread is golden and the cheese is melted.

5. While the sandwiches cook, reheat the soup in a medium saucepan over medium-high heat.

6. Slice each sandwich into 4 sticks for dipping and serve them with the hot soup.

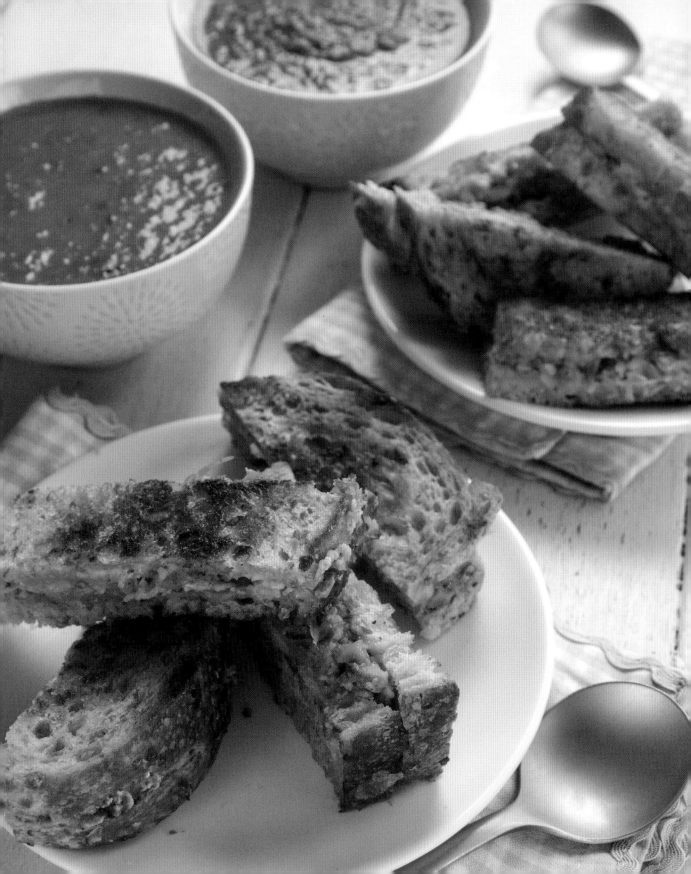

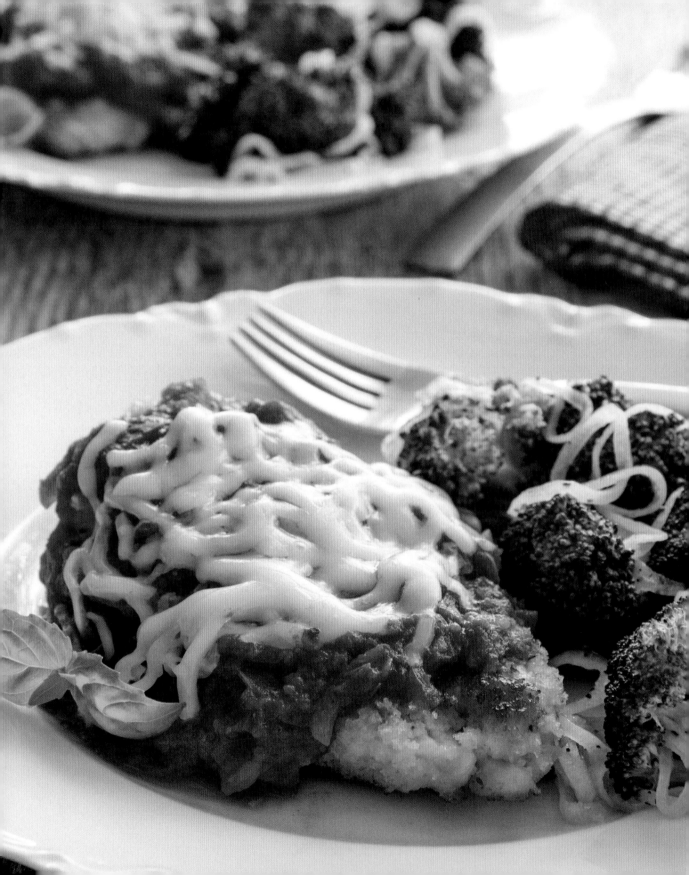

Skinny Chicken Parmesan with Roasted Broccoli

This protein-packed meal is fast, easy, and great for busy weeknights. I skip some of the more tedious chicken Parm steps like flattening the chicken; you save time and calories, since the chicken needs fewer bread crumbs to cover it. P.S. Broccoli covered in marinara sauce is the best thing ever . . . try it!

Makes 4 servings | Serving size: 1 chicken breast and about 1/3 cup cooked broccoli
Per serving: calories 370; fat 8 g; saturated fat 3 g; fiber 4 g; protein 38 g; carbohydrates 35 g;
sugar 6.5 g | Prep time: 10 minutes | Cook time: 30 minutes

2 cups broccoli florets
3 garlic cloves, thinly sliced
1 small yellow onion, sliced into rings
Olive oil spray
Kosher salt and freshly ground black pepper
4 boneless, skinless chicken breasts
¾ cup panko bread crumbs
2 tablespoons freshly grated Parmesan cheese
1 teaspoon garlic powder
1 egg
1 cup marinara sauce (see page 155), plus more for dipping if you like
½ cup shredded mozzarella cheese

1. Preheat the oven to 425°F.

2. Place the broccoli, garlic, and onion in a 9 × 9-inch casserole dish. Give it a shot of oil spray and a pinch each of salt and pepper, and toss. Roast for 25 minutes, tossing once halfway through cooking.

3. Meanwhile, in a pie pan or large shallow bowl, mix together the panko bread crumbs, Parmesan, and garlic powder. In another pie pan or shallow bowl, whisk the egg.

4. Spray a large skillet with oil spray and place over medium-high heat.

5. Working with one at a time, dunk a chicken breast in the egg, then the bread crumb mixture, and place it in the hot skillet. Cook for 10 minutes on each side, or until golden brown.

6. Transfer the chicken to a rimmed baking sheet, top with the marinara sauce and mozzarella, and bake for 10 minutes, or until the cheese is melted and the chicken is cooked through (no pink on the inside and the juices run clear).

7. Serve the chicken and broccoli with more marinara sauce if you like. I enjoy dipping my broccoli in it—yum!

Spinach and Goat Cheese Chicken Sandwiches and Garlic French Fries

A popular burger chain known for smashing its burgers makes one of my favorite chicken sandwiches, so of course I had to try to re-create it at home, and though I skip the "smashing" of the chicken (just too labor-intensive), I think it's spot-on!

These yummy garlic fries will be an instant hit, so go ahead and dog-ear the page so you can come back and make them anytime you crave some French fries. Trust me, you'll be glad you did it.

Makes 4 servings | Serving size: 1 sandwich and about ⅔ cup fries | Per serving: calories 398; fat 12 g; saturated fat 3 g; fiber 7 g; protein 27 g; carbohydrates 59.5 g; sugar 6 g
Prep time: 20 minutes | Cook time: 25 minutes

POTATOES
4 medium russet potatoes
1 teaspoon kosher salt
1 tablespoon olive oil
5 garlic cloves, unpeeled

CHICKEN SANDWICHES
2 boneless, skinless chicken breasts
2 teaspoons olive oil
Kosher salt and freshly ground black pepper
1 tablespoon balsamic vinegar
1 garlic clove, minced
1 tablespoon fresh lemon juice
4 whole wheat burger buns
½ cucumber, cut into ⅛-inch-thick slices
2 tablespoons crumbled goat cheese
¾ cup baby spinach
4 red onion slices
1 tomato, cut into ¼-inch-thick slices

1. Preheat the oven to 425°F. Line two rimmed baking sheets with parchment paper.

2. Make the fries: Peel the potatoes and cut them into ¼-inch-thick sticks, adding them to a large bowl as you work. Sprinkle with salt, drizzle with oil, and toss. Spread the potatoes on the prepared baking sheets, add the garlic cloves, and roast for 25 minutes, flipping once halfway through.

3. Meanwhile, make the chicken: Cut the chicken breasts in half horizontally by placing the palm of your hand on the top of a breast and using a sharp small knife to carefully cut all the way around and through, leaving you with 2 thin cutlets from each breast.

4. Heat 1 teaspoon of the oil in a sauté pan over medium heat and add the chicken. Cook for 10 to 15 minutes total, flipping once, until cooked through (no pink on the inside and the juices run clear).

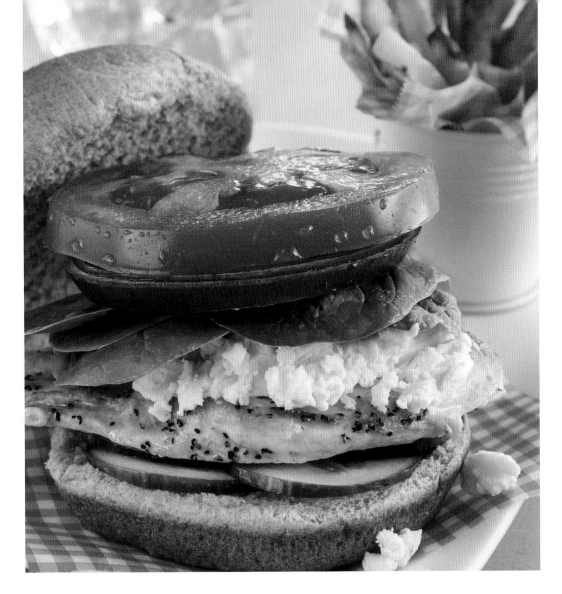

5. Meanwhile, in a small bowl, whisk together the remaining 1 teaspoon oil, the vinegar, garlic, and lemon juice. Set aside.

6. When the potatoes are done, carefully transfer the garlic cloves to a cutting board. Let them cool for a minute or two, then slice open, scrape out the soft garlic, and mince. Divide the fries among four plates and top with the roasted garlic.

7. To assemble the sandwiches, open each bun and add layers in this order: cucumber slices, chicken cutlet, ½ tablespoon goat cheese, spinach, drizzle of the vinaigrette, onion, tomato, top of the bun. Serve on the plates alongside the fries.

Chicken Lettuce Wraps

What if I told you that in less time than it would take to get into the car, drive to P.F. Chang's, and get a table, you could make these babies at home? Plus, mine are packed with veggies and loads of flavor, and you don't need to look for a parking spot.

So here's the deal—I make my own hoisin sauce. The stuff you buy from the store is packed with preservatives, fake dyes, and chemicals. Now, I know the thought of making your own may seem cumbersome, but you just add everything to a jar and shake it up! And if you're going through all the trouble to make the hoisin sauce (do you detect my sarcasm here?), you might as well make the Spicy Kung Pao Chicken for Two on page 187 this week!

Makes 4 servings | *Serving size: 10 chicken lettuce wraps* | *Per serving: calories 308; fat 13 g; saturated fat 0 g; fiber 4 g; protein 23 g; carbohydrates 25.5 g; sugar 8 g*
Prep time: 20 minutes | *Cook time: 15 minutes*

Olive oil spray
1 pound ground chicken
1 medium yellow onion, minced
1 cup minced white or other mushrooms
2 garlic cloves, minced
1 teaspoon grated peeled fresh ginger
2 tablespoons Homemade Hoisin Sauce (recipe follows)
1 tablespoon unseasoned rice wine vinegar
¼ teaspoon red pepper flakes (optional)
1 (8-ounce) can water chestnuts, drained and diced
2 green onions, thinly sliced
2 carrots, grated
1 head butter lettuce

1. Spray a large sauté pan with oil spray and place over medium-high heat. Add the chicken and cook for 5 minutes, crumbling the chicken as you work.

2. Add the onion and mushrooms to the pan and cook for 5 minutes, stirring a couple times to avoid burning and to help the chicken cook. Add the garlic, ginger, hoisin sauce, vinegar, and red pepper flakes (if using) and cook for 2 minutes, mixing well to distribute the sauce evenly.

3. Add the water chestnuts, green onions, and carrots and cook for 2 minutes. Cover the pan, turn off the heat, and let sit for 5 minutes.

4. To serve, scoop the chicken mixture into the lettuce leaves, fold up, and devour.

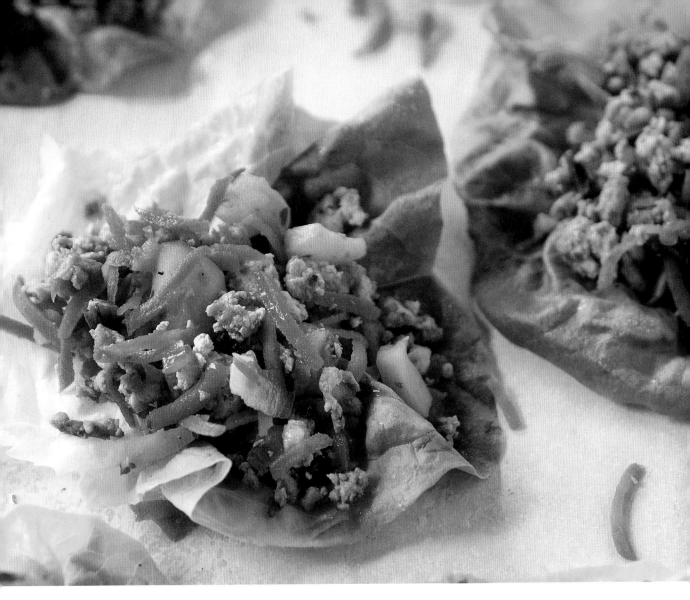

Homemade Hoisin Sauce

Makes ½ cup

½ cup reduced-sodium soy sauce

2 tablespoons all-natural peanut butter

1 tablespoon honey

2 teaspoons unseasoned rice vinegar

2 teaspoons toasted sesame oil

1 garlic clove, grated or minced

⅛ teaspoon freshly ground black pepper

1 teaspoon red miso paste

Place all the ingredients in a jar, cover, and shake well. Store in the refrigerator for up to 2 weeks.

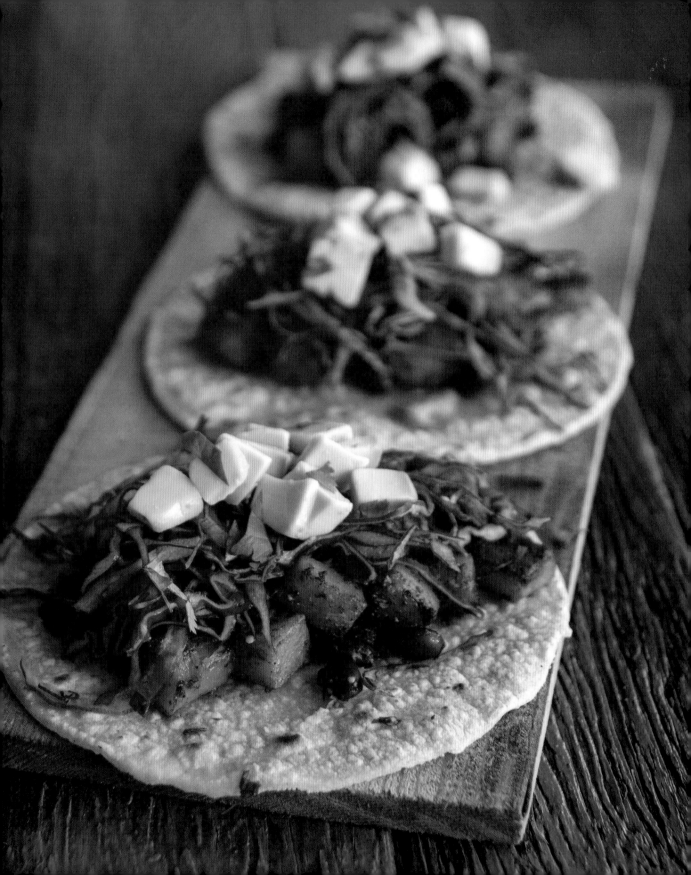

Black Bean and Butternut Squash Tacos

Vegan tacos for meat lovers! Honestly, I prefer these to all other tacos—they're so unique and packed full of flavor!

I first tried butternut squash tacos from a food truck in Southern California. There were three tacos to choose from—pork shoulder, chicken, and butternut squash—so naturally I got one of each. I was pleasantly surprised to find I enjoyed the vegan taco the best, and I've been making my own ever since. So try them out, and if you must have some animal protein in your tacos, add some shredded chicken.

Makes 4 servings | Serving size: 2 tacos | Per serving: calories 423; fat 15 g; saturated fat 3.5 g; fiber 12 g; protein 12 g; carbohydrates 65 g; sugar 4 g | Prep time: 10 minutes | Cook time: 25 minutes

TACOS
1 teaspoon olive oil
2 cups ¼-inch-cubed butternut squash
1 teaspoon chili powder
1 teaspoon garlic powder
½ teaspoon ground cumin
Kosher salt and freshly ground black pepper
1 (15-ounce) can black beans, drained and rinsed (preferably BPA-free cans)
8 (6-inch) whole wheat tortillas

SLAW
1 cup thinly sliced purple cabbage
¼ red onion, thinly sliced
3 tablespoons chopped fresh cilantro
1 tablespoon fresh lime juice
1 teaspoon olive oil
1 teaspoon red wine vinegar
Pinch of kosher salt
Pinch of freshly ground black pepper

TOPPINGS
1 avocado, diced
Chopped fresh cilantro (optional)
Hot sauce (optional)

1. Make the taco filling: Heat the oil in a large skillet over medium-high heat. Add the squash, chili powder, garlic powder, cumin, and salt and pepper to taste and toss together to coat. Cook, stirring often to avoid burning, until the squash is soft and slightly caramelized, 15 to 20 minutes. Add the beans and cook for 5 minutes or so to heat them up.

2. While the squash cooks, make the slaw: Place the cabbage, onion, cilantro, lime juice, oil, and vinegar in a medium bowl, add the salt and pepper, and toss.

3. Spread out the tortillas on one or two baking sheets and bake on your oven's lowest temperature (ideally 200°F) for 2 to 5 minutes, just until they're warm.

4. To assemble the tacos, spoon some taco filling onto each tortilla and top with slaw, avocado, and more cilantro (if you really love it like I do) and some of your favorite hot sauce (if you're feeling spicy). Dig in and enjoy—licking your fingers is fine, but try to avoid licking your plate.

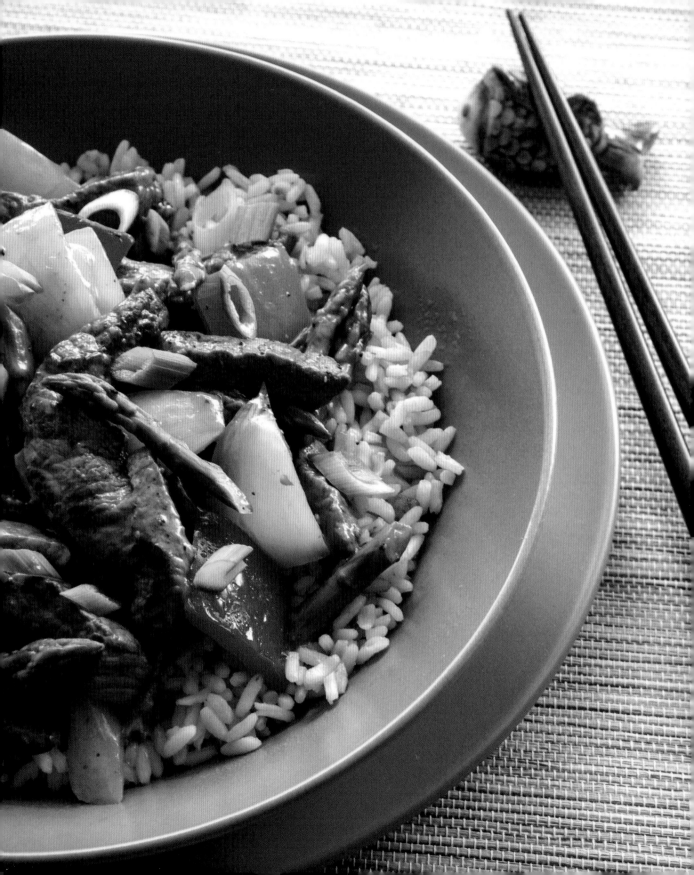

Pepper Steak with Asparagus and Brown Rice

I love asparagus. Not only is it delicious and easy to make, but it also goes so well with this pepper steak—the perfect addition to a very healthy meal.

Next time you're craving red meat, make this meal and watch your cravings melt away. Best of all, you'll feel fantastic after eating this healthy dish.

Makes 4 servings | *Serving size: about 1½ cups pepper steak and ¼ cup cooked rice*
Per serving: calories 415; fat 22 g; saturated fat 0.5 g; fiber 2 g; protein 33 g; carbohydrates 74 g; sugar 3 g
Prep time: 10 minutes | *Cook time: 20 minutes*

1 (1-pound) sirloin steak, cut into thin strips
3 garlic cloves, chopped
1 teaspoon red wine vinegar
1 teaspoon freshly ground black pepper
1 teaspoon reduced-sodium soy sauce
2 teaspoons toasted sesame oil
⅓ cup uncooked brown rice (you can also use cauliflower rice here!)
1 bunch asparagus, cut into bite-size pieces
1 red bell pepper, cut into bite-size pieces
1 medium yellow onion, cut into ½-inch pieces
2 teaspoons cornstarch

1. Place the steak strips, garlic, vinegar, pepper, soy sauce, and 1 teaspoon of the oil in a medium bowl or gallon-size freezer bag. Marinate for 10 minutes to 1 hour in the fridge (I marinate the steak while I cut the veggies).

2. In a small saucepan, stir together the rice and ⅔ cup water. Cover and bring to a low boil over medium heat, then turn the heat to low and cook, undisturbed, until all the liquid is absorbed, 15 to 20 minutes.

3. Meanwhile, in a large skillet over high heat, brown the steak strips in batches for 1 to 2 minutes. Reserve the marinade. Set the steak aside on a plate.

4. Turn the heat to medium-high and add the remaining 1 teaspoon oil to the skillet. Add the asparagus, bell pepper, onion, and reserved marinade, cover, and cook for 10 minutes, stirring two or three times to avoid burning.

5. In a small bowl, mix the cornstarch with ⅓ cup water. Add it to the veggies, stir, and cook over low heat for 5 minutes, or until the sauce has thickened.

6. Return the steak to the skillet and cook for 2 minutes to warm up. Serve over brown rice.

Chicken Apple Brie Quesadillas

There's this little bakery in my old town that makes amazing chicken-apple-Brie sandwiches, and to this day I simply call the bakery Chicken Apple Brie. When my friend Rachel first turned me on to this bakery's amazing sandwiches, we would text each other messages, like "Chicken Apple Brie, 1 p.m." and then we'd meet at the bakery to split a sandwich.

Well, when it came time to test this recipe I texted Rachel, "Chicken Apple Brie HELP," and she jumped into action, telling me what was memorable about the original. We've both moved away from that charming little town, but we agree that this quesadilla is a great stand-in—and without all that bread, you don't have to split it with anyone!

Makes 2 servings | Serving size: 1 quesadilla | Per serving: calories 458; fat 17 g; saturated fat 8 g; fiber 29 g; protein 30 g; carbohydrates 45 g; sugar 10 g | Prep time: 5 minutes | Cook time: 10 minutes

Olive oil spray
1 tablespoon 0% Greek yogurt
2 teaspoons Dijon mustard
½ teaspoon garlic powder
2 (10-inch) burrito-size whole wheat tortillas
4 tablespoons diced cold Brie cheese
1 Granny Smith apple, cored and sliced into matchsticks
1 cooked chicken breast, shredded (see page 132)
⅔ cup mixed greens

1. Lightly spray a large skillet with oil spray and place over medium-high heat.

2. In a small bowl, combine the yogurt, mustard, and garlic powder. Mix well and spread it on the tortillas.

3. Divide the Brie evenly between the tortillas and top with apple matchsticks and chicken. Fold the tortillas in half to make half-moon quesadillas.

4. Place the quesadillas in the hot skillet and toast for 5 minutes on each side, or until the cheese is melted and the tortillas are golden.

5. Transfer the quesadillas to a cutting board and open them up. Add half the greens to each, close the quesadillas, and use kitchen scissors to cut them into triangles. Serve hot.

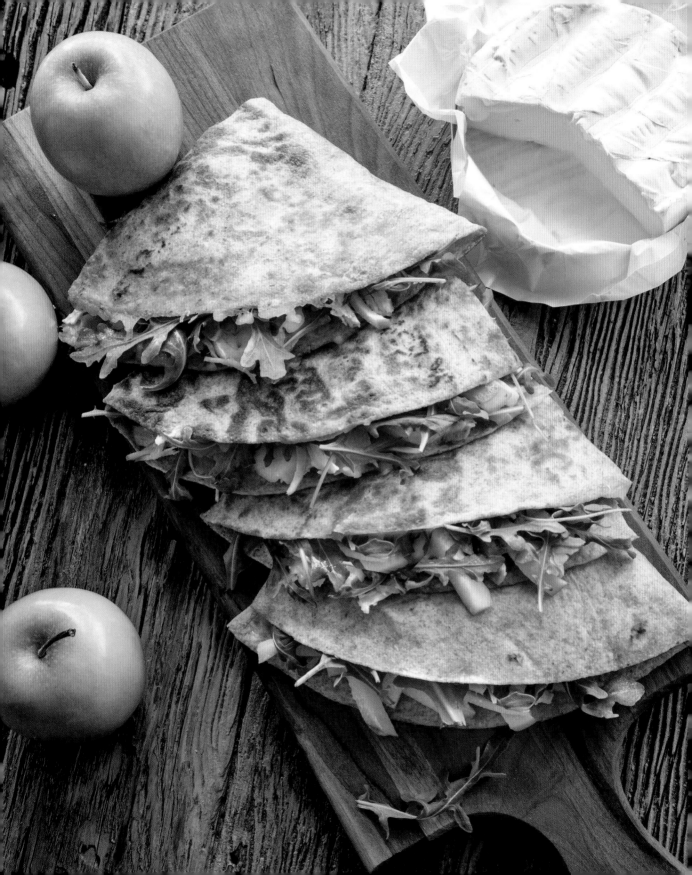

11

Date Night and Family Dinners on Detox Week

Here are some slightly fancier meals, the kind you make when you're trying to impress. Make them for your love for a homemade date night, to impress your in-laws, or just because you want to spoil your family (or yourself). They're all still easy, well . . . the Coq au Vin is intermediate.

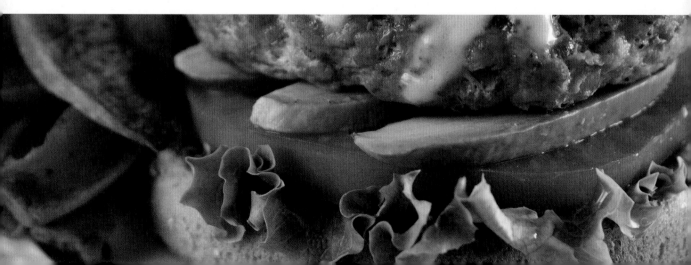

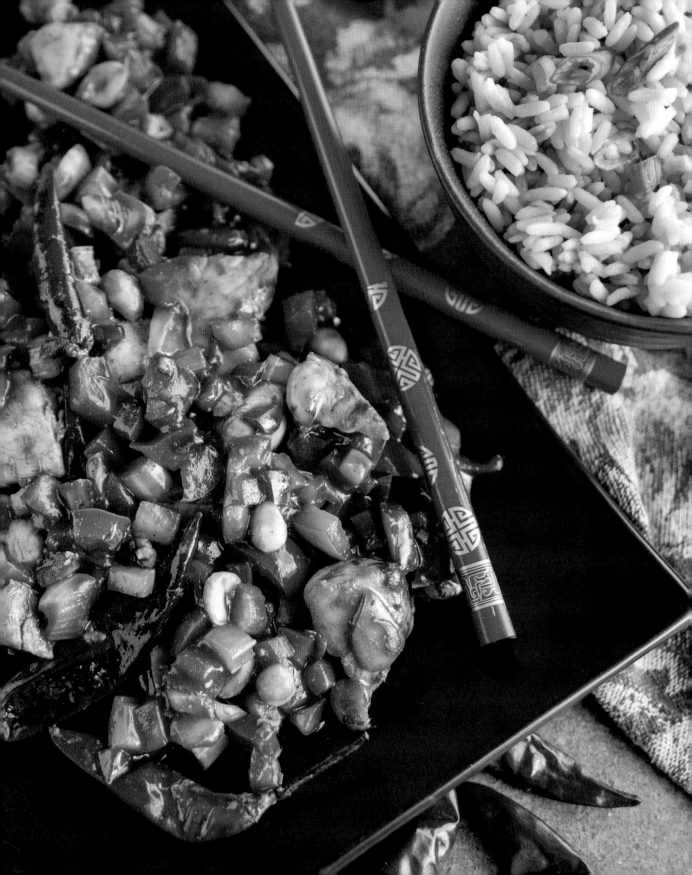

Spicy Kung Pao Chicken for Two

I love the movie *Grumpy Old Men*, and of course my favorite part is when Ann-Margret says she and her crush will be eating spicy food intentionally to keep them up . . . *all* . . . *night* . . . *long*.

I make this just for two, as it's way too spicy for my daughter, and honestly sometimes the parents just need to have their own special dinner. So feed the kids early, put them to bed, and make this for your spouse, crush, lover. It'll turn up the heat . . . all . . . night . . . long!

Makes 2 servings | Serving size: about 2¼ cups | Per serving: calories 418; fat 16.5 g; saturated fat 2.5 g; fiber 5 g; protein 35 g; carbohydrates 33 g; sugar 18 g
Prep time: 15 minutes | Cook time: 15 minutes

CHICKEN

2 chicken breasts, cut into ⅓-inch cubes
1 teaspoon reduced-sodium soy sauce
1 teaspoon unseasoned rice wine vinegar
½ teaspoon honey
½ teaspoon toasted sesame oil
½ teaspoon cornstarch

STIR-FRY

3 tablespoons reduced-sodium soy sauce
3 tablespoons balsamic vinegar
3 tablespoons Homemade Hoisin Sauce (page 177)
1 teaspoon raw organic sugar
1 teaspoon red pepper flakes
1 tablespoon cornstarch
½ teaspoon toasted sesame oil
5 to 10 dried red chiles (depending on your heat preference)
2 bell peppers (I like 1 red and 1 green), diced
3 celery stalks, diced
1 medium white or yellow onion, chopped in ¼-inch chunks
2 garlic cloves, minced
½ teaspoon grated peeled fresh ginger
¼ cup unsalted peanuts

1. Place all the chicken ingredients in a medium bowl or gallon-size freezer bag, mix well, and marinate in the fridge for at least 20 minutes or all day, if you have time.

2. Make the stir-fry: In a small bowl, whisk together the soy sauce, vinegar, hoisin sauce, sugar, red pepper flakes, and cornstarch. Mix well and set aside.

3. Heat the oil in a large skillet or wok over high heat, add the chiles, and cook for 1 minute, or until fragrant. Add the chicken and marinade and cook for 1 minute. Add the bell peppers, celery, and onion, lower the heat to medium-high, and cook for 5 minutes, stirring often to avoid burning.

4. Add the garlic, ginger, and peanuts, mix to combine, and cook for about 2 minutes, until the garlic is fragrant. Add the hoisin sauce mixture and cook for 1 to 2 minutes, until the chicken is cooked through and the sauce is thick.

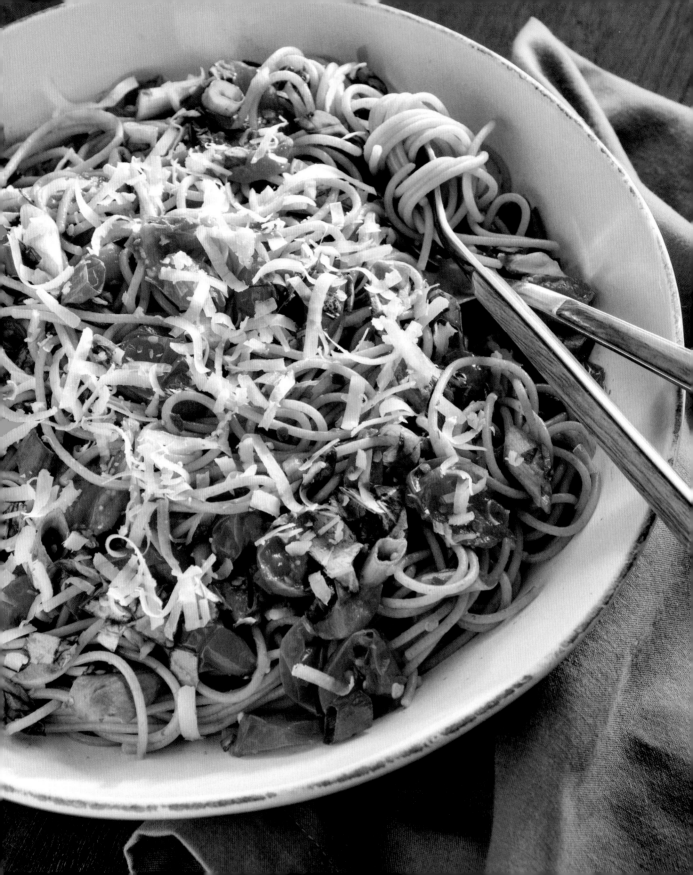

Bruschetta Pasta (. . . in Bed)

Ooh la la . . . we're getting a little sexy in this recipe. But honestly, you can eat this at a table—you don't have to go the naughty route (though I do recommend it). Hey, it's the Date Night chapter, right?

This meal for two can easily be doubled or tripled for the whole family, and speaking of family, my daughter loves it!

Makes 2 servings | Serving size: about 1¼ cups | Per serving: calories 302; fat 6 g; saturated fat 2 g; fiber 9 g; protein 14 g; carbohydrates 50 g; sugar 5 g | Prep time: 10 minutes | Cook time: 15 minutes

4 ounces spinach angel hair pasta (if you can't find spinach pasta, use whole wheat)
1 teaspoon olive oil
4 garlic cloves
10 ounces grape tomatoes, halved
Pinch of kosher salt
1½ cups fresh basil leaves, chopped
2 green onions, thinly sliced
½ to 2 teaspoons red pepper flakes (depending on your heat tolerance) (optional)
3 tablespoons freshly grated Parmesan cheese

1. Bring a large pot of water to a boil. Add the pasta and cook until al dente according to the package directions.

2. While the pasta is cooking, heat the oil in a large sauté pan over medium-low heat. Add the garlic, tomatoes, and salt and cook for 10 minutes, or until the tomatoes start to pop and cook down. Stir once or twice to avoid burning.

3. Drain the pasta, reserving ⅓ cup of the pasta water. Add the reserved pasta water to the tomatoes and simmer for about 5 minutes, until it's reduced into a sauce.

4. Turn off the heat, add the basil, green onions, red pepper flakes (if using), and pasta, and toss to coat the pasta in the sauce.

5. Serve in a large bowl, top with cheese, and feed each other from the same fork in bed. . . . Or serve on two plates and curl up on the couch.

One-Pan Roasted Chicken with Root Veggies

If there was one thing I could cook every single day of my life, it would be a whole chicken. I find so much joy in the process and the result, and I *know* that no matter what is going wrong in my life I can always roast a perfect chicken. Follow these directions and you, too, can make the perfect roasted chicken. I kept this recipe easy—no trussing, no fancy stuffing, just easy-peasy—so try it out and wow your family with your superb kitchen skills.

Makes 8 servings | Serving size: 4 ounces chicken and ⅔ cup veggies | Per serving: calories 378; fat 19 g; saturated fat 5 g; fiber 3 g; protein 24 g; carbohydrates 23 g; sugar 2 g
Prep time: 15 minutes | Cook time: 2 hours 15 minutes

MARINADE
1 tablespoon olive oil
Juice of 1 lemon (reserve the juiced halves)
1 teaspoon chili powder
1 teaspoon paprika
1 tablespoon garlic powder
½ teaspoon kosher salt
½ teaspoon freshly ground black pepper

CHICKEN AND VEGETABLES
1 (5-to-7-pound) chicken
6 garlic cloves, smashed with the back of a knife or fork (you don't even need to peel them!)
2 carrots, cut into 1-inch pieces
5 small Yukon Gold potatoes, quartered
1 large parsnip, peeled and cut into 1-inch pieces

1. Preheat the oven to 350°F.

2. In a small bowl, whisk together the marinade ingredients. Set aside.

3. Remove the neck and giblets from the chicken and discard (or reserve them to make chicken broth). Add the reserved lemon halves and garlic cloves to the chicken cavity.

4. Place the chicken in the center of a large roasting pan and arrange the carrots, potatoes, and parsnip around it.

5. Pour half the marinade over the chicken and the other half over the vegetables. Roast for about 2 hours, basting the chicken and the veggies two or three times. The chicken is done when the internal temperature is 165°F (stick the thermometer into the thickest part of the breast) and the juices run clear.

6. Transfer the chicken to a carving board or rimmed baking sheet to rest. Mix the veggies in the pan juices, crank up the oven to 425°F, and roast for 15 minutes while the chicken rests. Use a wooden spoon to toss the veggies a couple times while they cook.

7. Carve the chicken into 10 pieces: 2 legs, 2 thighs, and 2 wings, and cut each chicken breast in half to make 4 breast portions. Serve with the yummy roasted veggies.

Citrus-Glazed Salmon with Sesame Broccoli

Okay, ladies, let's talk about how great salmon is for our bodies! First off, when you're crampy and bloated and feel like your body is betraying you one week a month, eat salmon! It's packed so full of vitamin B_{12} and omega-3s that you'll be feeling better fast . . . and looking better, too! Salmon is a great beauty food, so if you break out during that dreaded week, salmon will help.

Makes 4 servings | Serving size: 4 ounces salmon and about 1 cup broccoli
Per serving: calories 322; fat 17 g; saturated fat 3's g; fiber 3 g; protein 26 g;
carbohydrates 19 g; sugar 12 g | Prep time: 5 minutes | Cook time: 55 minutes

---

SALMON
Juice of 2 oranges
2 tablespoons orange marmalade
2 tablespoons reduced-sodium soy sauce
1 tablespoon rice wine vinegar
2 garlic cloves, grated or minced
½ cup chicken broth
1 teaspoon pure maple syrup
1 (1-pound) salmon fillet, cut into 4 pieces

BROCCOLI
4 cups broccoli florets
1 tablespoon sesame seeds
1 tablespoon toasted sesame oil
1 tablespoon reduced-sodium soy sauce

1. Preheat the oven to 350°F.

2. Make the salmon: Place the orange juice, marmalade, soy sauce, rice wine vinegar, garlic, chicken broth, and maple syrup in a small saucepan. Bring to a boil over medium-high heat, then reduce the heat to a simmer and cook for 20 minutes, stirring often to avoid burning. Place the salmon fillets in a 9 × 13-inch baking dish. When the glaze has reduced by half, about 10 minutes, pour half of the glaze over the salmon fillets. Reserve the remaining glaze.

3. Make the broccoli: In a second 9 × 13-inch casserole dish, toss together the broccoli, sesame seeds, oil, and soy sauce until the broccoli is well coated. Roast the broccoli for about 15 minutes, until it starts to soften. Give it another stir, and return it to the oven along with the dish of salmon. Roast for 10 minutes, then pour the remaining glaze over the salmon. Roast both the broccoli and the salmon for 10 minutes more, or until the broccoli is tender and the salmon flakes when pierced with a fork, then serve.

Veggie-Packed Coq au Vin

So, I have to admit that I was a little worried that I would be struck down by lightning when I swapped in turkey bacon for pork bacon in a coq au vin recipe. I survived unscathed and was happy to find that I couldn't tell the difference. I also used lemon juice in place of the brandy (there's wine in here, so the chicken is drunk enough). I always add lemon juice at the end, so I figured why not use it to deglaze the pan—and another skinny hack was born in this dish!

I've been diligent about making very easy meals for this book, and this is the exception. There's a lot going on, but just follow the instructions step by step and you, too, can master this amazing French dish. You'll need a Dutch oven or a large lidded skillet that you can move from the stovetop to the oven.

Makes 4 servings | Serving size: one chicken thigh and about ½ cup vegetables
Per serving: calories 499; fat 18 g; saturated fat 8 g; fiber 4 g; protein 41 g;
carbohydrates 18.5 g; sugar 8 g | Prep time: 15 minutes | Cook time: 1 hour 45 minutes

3 slices turkey bacon, sliced into ¼ inch pieces

2 teaspoons olive oil

4 bone-in chicken thighs

1 medium yellow onion, halved and sliced into thin half-moons

5 carrots, cut into 1-inch diagonal chunks

Kosher salt

1 garlic clove, minced

2 tablespoons fresh lemon juice

1 cup chicken broth

½ cup dry red wine

10 thyme sprigs

8 ounces white mushrooms, sliced (about 1½ cups)

1 tablespoon unsalted butter

1 tablespoon all-purpose flour

½ cup frozen pearl onions

1. Preheat the oven to 250°F.

2. Heat a Dutch oven or large ovenproof skillet over medium heat. Add the turkey bacon and 1 teaspoon of the oil and cook until the bacon starts to brown, about 5 minutes. Transfer the bacon to a plate and add the chicken thighs to the pan, skin side down. Brown for 10 minutes, then transfer the thighs to the plate with the bacon. Place the onion and carrots in the Dutch oven and add a pinch of salt. Sauté until the onion starts to brown and soften, about 15 minutes. Add the garlic and cook for 1 minute.

3. Add the lemon juice and scrape the bottom of the pan to loosen any browned bits. Return the chicken and turkey bacon to the pan and add the broth and wine. Top with the thyme sprigs and bring to a simmer.

4. Cover the pan and place it in the oven. Cook for 1 hour 20 minutes, turning the chicken thighs over halfway through.

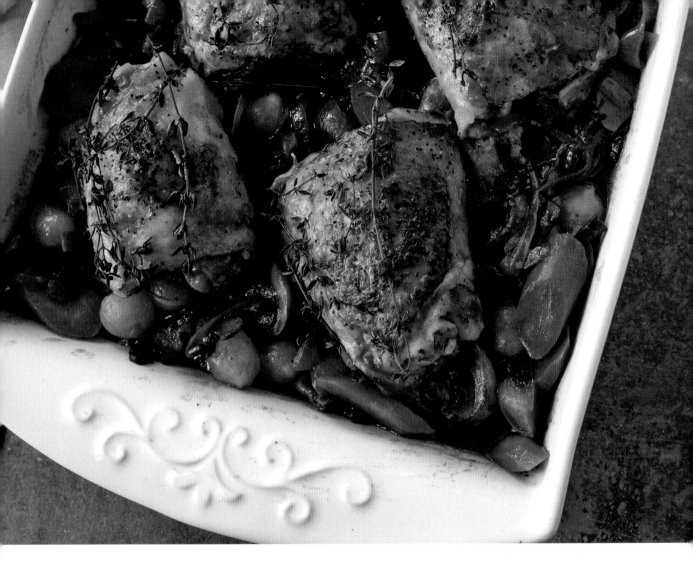

5. Meanwhile, heat the remaining 1 teaspoon oil in a large skillet over medium heat. Add the mushrooms and cook, stirring occasionally, until browned, about 5 minutes.

6. Push the mushrooms to one side of the skillet and melt the butter on the other side. Add the flour to the butter and whisk together with a wooden spoon for about 5 minutes, until you have a lightly browned paste (this is a roux). Add the pearl onions and stir to combine the onions, mushrooms, and roux. Set aside until the chicken is done.

7. Remove the chicken from the oven and set the Dutch oven back on the stovetop. Transfer the chicken to a plate while you thicken up the sauce.

8. Add the mushrooms and onions to the Dutch oven with the sauce and turn the heat to medium, stirring to avoid burning. When the sauce is thick enough to coat the back of a spoon, about 30 minutes, return the chicken to the pan and spoon some sauce over it. Serve hot! This is even better on the second day, so make extra if you love leftovers.

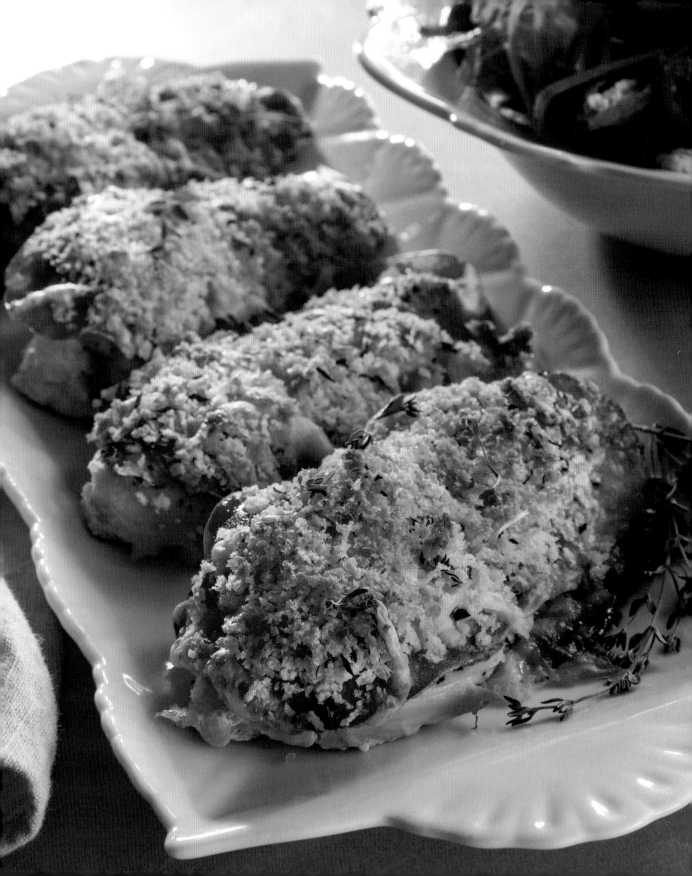

Easy Chicken Cordon Bleu with French Bistro Salad

A few years ago I spent a long vacation in Paris, and avid salad fan that I am, I always ordered salad with my French bistro *déjeuners* (lunches). Every single time, I was served a lovely house salad with a dressing that looked like ranch, but tasted like a mild horseradish . . . which may sound strange, but it's amazing! You need this salad dressing in your life, so don't skip it—plus, you and I both know that the French know what they're doing when it comes to food.
Bon appétit!

Makes 4 servings | Serving size: 1 chicken breast and about ⅓ cup salad | Per serving: calories 309; fat 9 g; saturated fat 3.5 g; fiber 4 g; protein 40 g; carbohydrates 17 g; sugar 4.5 g
Prep time: 15 minutes | Cook time: 25 minutes

Olive oil spray
4 boneless, skinless chicken breasts
2 teaspoons Dijon mustard
4 slices prosciutto
½ cup shredded Gruyère or provolone cheese
½ cup panko bread crumbs
1 teaspoon chopped fresh thyme

SALAD
⅓ cup 0% Greek yogurt
1 tablespoon unsweetened almond milk (but any milk will work)
1 tablespoon prepared horseradish
1½ teaspoons chopped fresh dill
¾ teaspoon chopped fresh thyme
Kosher salt and freshly ground black pepper
2 romaine hearts
½ cup halved cherry tomatoes
1 carrot, grated
⅓ cup cucumber slices

1. Preheat the oven to 450°F. Spray a 9 × 13-inch baking dish with oil spray.

2. Arrange the chicken breasts in the baking dish so that they don't touch. Smear the top of each with ½ teaspoon of the mustard and top each with a slice of prosciutto, 2 tablespoons of the shredded cheese, and 2 tablespoons of the panko. Sprinkle the thyme over the chicken breasts, spray lightly with oil spray, and bake for 20 to 25 minutes, until the cheese is melted, the panko is browned, and the chicken reaches an internal temperature of 165°F and the juices run clear.

3. Meanwhile, make the salad: In a small bowl, combine the yogurt, almond milk, horseradish, dill, thyme, and salt and pepper to taste. Mix well and set aside.

4. Cut the romaine into bite-size pieces and divide among the plates. Top with the tomatoes, carrot, and cucumber. Drizzle the salad dressing on top, and serve with the chicken.

Tuscan Sun Chicken with Broccoli and Potato Casserole

Here's the skinny on this little ditty: I tested this marinade on every single cut of chicken, and I couldn't figure out which I liked best! So instead of choosing just one, see Chicken Roasting Times for all the cuts, so you can get your favorite (or what's on sale) and choose for yourself.

Makes 4 servings | Serving size: 4 ounces chicken breast or 1 thigh or 2 legs/wings and 1 cup vegetables | Per serving: calories 495; fat 24.5 g; saturated fat 1 g; fiber 6 g; protein 28 g; carbohydrates 42 g; sugar 3 g | Prep time: 10 minutes | Cook time: 1 to 2 hours (see Chicken Roasting Times)

CHICKEN
1 tablespoon olive oil
Zest and juice of 1 lemon
1 tablespoon garlic powder
4 garlic cloves, gently smashed
Pinch of kosher salt
Pinch of freshly ground black pepper
4 portions of chicken (2 halved chicken breasts, 4 thighs, or 8 chicken legs or wings)

BROCCOLI AND POTATO CASSEROLE
4 medium Yukon Gold potatoes, each cut into 6 half-moons
1 tablespoon olive oil
1 teaspoon garlic powder
1 teaspoon paprika
1 teaspoon chili powder
Pinch of kosher salt
Pinch of freshly ground black pepper
3½ cups chopped broccoli florets
1 green onion, thinly sliced

1. Make the chicken: Place the lemon zest and juice, garlic powder, garlic, salt, and pepper in a gallon-size freezer bag and seal the bag. Squish around to mix, then add the chicken and shake to coat well. Place in the fridge to marinate for at least 1 hour or up to 12 hours.

2. Preheat the oven to 350°F.

3. Roast the chicken (see Chicken Roasting Times).

4. Make the casserole: Place the potatoes, oil, garlic powder, paprika, chili powder, salt, and pepper in a 9 × 13-inch casserole dish and mix to coat the potatoes. Roast the potatoes for 30 minutes, shaking and flipping a few times to avoid sticking. Add the broccoli, toss, and roast for another 30 minutes, or until the potatoes are tender when poked with a fork and the broccoli is browned and slightly softened.

5. Serve the chicken with the casserole.

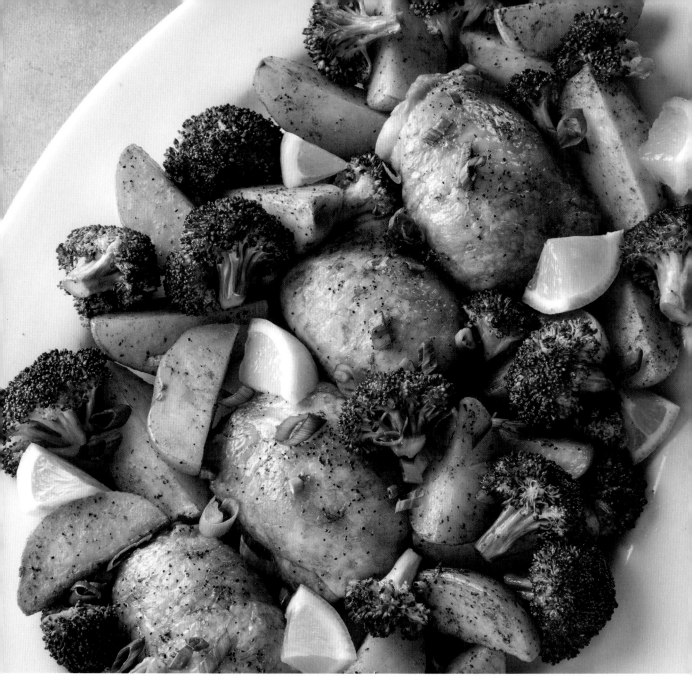

CHICKEN ROASTING TIMES

- Whole chicken: 350°F for 2 hours (will yield 8 portions)
- Legs and thighs: 350°F for 45 minutes
- Wings: 350°F for 30 minutes
- Bone-in breast: 350°F for 40 minutes

Avocado Club Cheeseburgers with Sweet Potato Fries

I know that the recipe name is a little deceitful since the recipe calls for turkey and not beef, so as a peace offering, here's a recommendation: Take this opportunity to try out bison! It tastes just like beef and has fewer calories, less fat, and more nutrients than beef. It will be your new favorite red meat!

Try this with ground turkey first, though. You can hardly tell it's a turkey burger with all the toppings, plus it has less fat and calories than beef!

Makes 4 servings | Serving size: 1 burger and about 1 cup fries | Per serving: calories 477; fat 22.5 g; saturated fat 8 g; fiber 5 g; protein 39 g; carbohydrates 39.5 g; sugar 9 g
Prep time: 15 minutes | Cook time: 45 minutes

SWEET POTATO FRIES
3 medium sweet potatoes
1 tablespoon olive oil
1 teaspoon garlic salt
½ teaspoon freshly ground black pepper

SAUCE
2 tablespoons Dijon mustard
⅓ cup 0% Greek yogurt
1 garlic clove, minced
Kosher salt and freshly ground black pepper

CHEESEBURGERS
Olive oil spray
4 slices turkey bacon, halved
1 package ground turkey
¼ cup minced red onion
1 garlic clove, minced
Pinch of kosher salt
Pinch of freshly ground black pepper
¼ cup grated sharp cheddar cheese
4 whole wheat burger buns
½ avocado
4 romaine leaves, halved
1 large tomato, cut into 4 thick slices

1. Make the fries: Preheat the oven to 375°F. Line two rimmed baking sheets with parchment paper.

2. Peel the sweet potatoes and cut them into steak fry–size wedges, tossing them into a large bowl as you work. Add the oil, garlic salt, and pepper and toss to coat the fries. Spread out the fries evenly on the prepared baking sheets and bake for 45 minutes, flipping halfway through.

3. Make the sauce: Whisk together all the sauce ingredients in a small bowl. Set aside to let the flavors blend.

4. Make the burgers: Line a plate with paper towels. Heat a large sauté pan over medium heat, spray with oil spray, add the turkey bacon, and brown to your liking. Transfer to the prepared plate, leaving the oil and drippings in the pan.

5. In a medium bowl, mix together with your clean hands the ground turkey, onion, garlic, kosher salt, and pepper until just

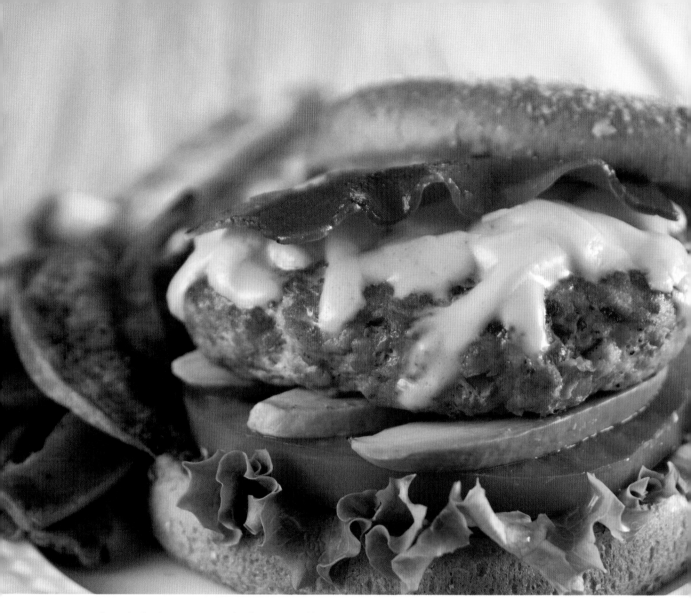

combined; don't overmix or the burgers will be tough. Form into 4 patties and make a little dimple in the center of each so that they keep their shape.

6. With the pan from the bacon over medium-low heat, add the patties and cook for 8 minutes, undisturbed. Flip, top each patty with cheese, and cook for 8 minutes, until cooked through with no pink in the center.

7. Place the bottom buns on four plates and layer each of them as follows: romaine, tomato, avocado, burger, bacon. Smear the top buns with sauce, then top the burgers. Divide the fries among the plates alongside the burgers and serve.

Oven-Fried Parmesan Pork Chops with a Crisp Green Salad

This recipe is inspired by the fried pork chops in my first cookbook, *Lose Weight by Eating*. But in my defense, I cut even more calories in this version, and, well ... I love fried pork chops.

In the first recipe, I fried the pork chops on the stovetop in very little oil, but when I moved to frigid (well, in comparison to California) Idaho, I started looking for any reason to turn on the oven. On a particularly cold night (I think it was 9°F outside) I finally hit the sweet spot on this recipe. So if it's the heat of the summer, use the recipe in the first book, and if it's cold out, here you go.

Makes 4 servings | Serving size: 1 pork chop and 1 cup salad | Per serving: calories 227; fat 5 g; saturated fat 2 g; fiber 1 g; protein 32 g; carbohydrates 11.5 g; sugar 4 g
Prep time: 10 minutes | Cook time: 20 minutes

CREAMY HONEY-MUSTARD DRESSING

1 tablespoon Dijon mustard

1½ teaspoons honey

¼ cup 0% Greek yogurt

2 tablespoons 2% milk (any milk will work)

½ teaspoon garlic powder

Kosher salt and freshly ground black pepper

PORK CHOPS

Olive oil spray

⅓ cup panko bread crumbs

3 tablespoons freshly grated Parmesan cheese

1 teaspoon garlic powder

⅛ teaspoon kosher salt

⅛ teaspoon freshly ground black pepper

1 egg

4 bone-in pork chops, fat trimmed off

SALAD

4 cups baby spinach

½ red bell pepper, cut into strips

¼ cup ¼-inch-diced cucumber

1 green onion, thinly sliced

1. Make the pork chops: Place all the dressing ingredients in a mason jar with a tight-fitting lid or small bowl, cover, and shake or whisk vigorously. Set aside to let the flavors blend.

2. Preheat the oven to 425°F and spray a rimmed baking sheet with oil spray.

3. In a pie pan or large shallow bowl, mix together the bread crumbs, cheese, garlic powder, salt, and pepper.

4. In a second pie pan or large shallow bowl, whisk the egg.

5. One by one, dip the pork chops into the egg, then the bread crumbs, coating them completely. Transfer the coated pork chops to the prepared baking sheet.

6. Spray the tops of the pork chops lightly with oil spray, then bake for 10 minutes. Flip the pork chops and bake for 10 minutes more, or until they are firm and cooked through (no pink on the inside).

7. Make the salad: Place the spinach, bell pepper, cucumber, and green onion in a large bowl, top with the dressing, and toss well.

8. To serve, I like to place the salad in the center of the plate and top it with the pork chop, though this dish is equally delicious if you serve them side by side.

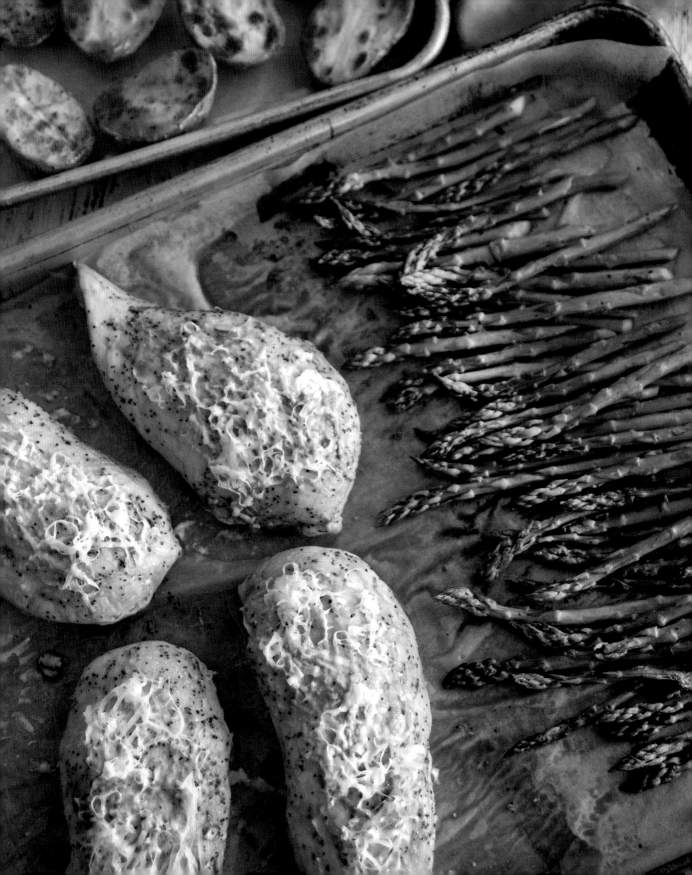

Two-Sheet-Pan Chicken and Veggies

Have you seen those popular sheet-pan recipes? I love the idea of cooking all your food on a single sheet pan—the cleanup is a breeze. My only issue is that you can't really fit *that much* food on a single sheet pan—so this is a two-sheet-pan recipe. You'll be hungry, and we want you satisfied!

Makes 4 servings | Serving size: 1 chicken breast and about 1 cup veggies
Per serving: calories 355; fat 7 g; saturated fat 2 g; fiber 16 g; protein 34 g;
carbohydrates 38 g; sugar 2 g | Prep time: 15 minutes | Cook time: 65 minutes

---

SHEET PAN #1

4 Yukon Gold potatoes, cut into bite-size chunks
1 teaspoon olive oil
½ teaspoon garlic powder
⅛ teaspoon kosher salt
⅛ teaspoon freshly ground black pepper

SHEET PAN #2

1 bunch asparagus, ends trimmed
4 boneless, skinless chicken breasts
1 teaspoon olive oil
Kosher salt and freshly ground black pepper
1 tablespoon Dijon mustard
1 garlic clove, finely chopped, or 1 teaspoon
   garlic powder
2 tablespoons grated Gruyère cheese

1. Position one oven rack in the middle of the oven and the second rack one spot below. Preheat the oven to 350°F. Line two rimmed baking sheets with parchment paper.

2. Spread out the potatoes on one baking sheet, drizzle the oil on top, and sprinkle with the garlic powder, salt, and pepper. Bake for 30 minutes, tossing once halfway through.

3. On the other baking sheet, arrange the asparagus on one side and the chicken breasts on the other. Drizzle ½ teaspoon of the oil over the asparagus and sprinkle with a pinch each of salt and pepper.

4. In a small bowl, combine the remaining ½ teaspoon oil, the mustard, and garlic. Spread the mixture over the chicken.

5. Set the second sheet in the oven and bake for 30 minutes (while you have the oven open, give the potatoes another toss and leave them in there—they need a full hour).

6. Remove both sheets from the oven, divide the asparagus among four plates, and top the chicken breasts with the Gruyère. Place under the broiler for 2 to 3 minutes, until the cheese is bubbling, watching closely to avoid burning. While the chicken is under the broiler, plate the potatoes.

7. Place a chicken breast on each plate alongside the potatoes. Cleanup is easy: Simply toss out the parchment paper and move the baking sheets to the dishwasher . . . no scrubbing needed, hurray!

Teriyaki Turkey Burgers
with Potato Salad

Originally I wanted to put this in the 30-minute meals section, and technically you can make it in 30 minutes—but it would be a very hectic half hour, so I moved it here. Life is stressful enough—dinner shouldn't be, too!

This potato salad is so yummy and unique! Living in Idaho, I get to try all kinds of amazing potato dishes, and this potato salad is my version of one of them—instead of a heavy mayo base, this has a lighter vinegar-and-mustard base.

Makes 4 servings | Serving size: 1 turkey burger and about ⅔ cup potato salad
Per serving: calories 272; fat 12 g; saturated fat 5 g; fiber 6 g; protein 19 g;
carbohydrates 58 g; sugar 14 g | Prep time: 20 minutes | Cook time: 30 minutes

POTATO SALAD
1 pound Yukon Gold potatoes
2 tablespoons fresh lemon juice
1 tablespoon grainy mustard
1 teaspoon apple cider vinegar
1 celery stalk, thinly sliced
1 green onion, thinly sliced
2 tablespoons chopped fresh flat-leaf parsley

TERIYAKI SAUCE
2 tablespoons reduced-sodium soy sauce
1 tablespoon unseasoned rice wine vinegar
½ garlic clove, grated
½ teaspoon grated peeled fresh ginger
3 tablespoons finely chopped fresh pineapple
1 teaspoon cornstarch
1 teaspoon honey

TURKEY BURGERS
1 pound ground turkey
Dash of reduced-sodium soy sauce
1 egg
2 tablespoons bread crumbs

1 garlic clove, grated
Olive oil spray
4 slices fresh pineapple
4 slices provolone cheese
4 whole wheat burger buns
4 romaine leaves, halved
4 slices tomato
4 red onion slices

1. Make the potato salad: Fill a saucepan two-thirds full of water and set it next to a cutting board.

2. Cut the potatoes into bite-size chunks, placing them in the water as you go. (I like to leave the skins on; it holds them together better.) Bring the water to a boil over medium-high heat and cook the potatoes for 10 to 15 minutes, until soft when pierced with a fork. Reserve 1 cup of the potato cooking water and set aside. Drain the potatoes and let them cool for 15 minutes.

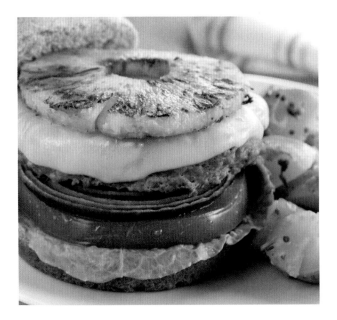

3. While the potatoes are cooking, in a small bowl, whisk together the lemon juice, mustard, and vinegar. Add the dressing and ½ cup of the reserved potato cooking water to the pot of drained potatoes. Mix well and let the dressing soak in for 5 minutes, adding more potato cooking water as needed if the potatoes are a little dry. Transfer the potato salad to the fridge to cool, or serve at room temperature. (You can make the potato salad the day before—it gets better as it sits.)

4. Make the teriyaki sauce: Place all the sauce ingredients and 2 tablespoons water in a small saucepan over medium heat and cook for about 5 minutes, until thick. Set aside.

5. Make the burgers: In a medium bowl, use your clean hands to mix together the turkey, soy sauce, egg, bread crumbs, and garlic until just combined; don't overmix or the burgers will be tough. Form 4 large, thin patties (they will shrink, so make them really flat and really big!).

6. Heat a large sauté pan over medium heat, lightly spray it with oil spray, and cook the pineapple rings for 5 to 8 minutes on each side, until soft and caramelized. Set aside. Spray the pan with a little more oil and add the turkey patties. Cook for 5 to 8 minutes on each side, until they're cooked through (no pink on the inside). Top with the provolone in the last 3 minutes.

7. Place the bottom buns on four plates and layer each of them in the following order: romaine, tomato, onion, burger. Spoon some of the teriyaki sauce over the patties and top with the cooked pineapple and top bun. Divide the potato salad among the plates alongside the burgers and serve.

Chicken Potpie Pasta

I know, right? . . . This sounds amazing! It is, and it is surprisingly easy to make! For all my vegetarian friends, you can easily make this meatless by using vegetable broth in place of chicken broth and using more veggies in place of the chicken, and, if desired, adding 1 cup cubed, crumbled tofu.

This is one of those meals that you can make right out of the pantry and freezer! Box of pasta, check . . . frozen veggies, check . . . and you probably have milk and maybe even some leftover cooked chicken breast stashed in your fridge.

Makes 6 servings | Serving size: about 1 cup | Per serving: calories 481; fat 11 g; saturated fat 5 g; fiber 8 g; protein 26 g; carbohydrates 71 g; sugar 9.5 g | Prep time: 5 minutes | Cook time: 40 minutes

1 box whole wheat penne pasta

TOPPING
2 tablespoons freshly grated Parmesan cheese
2 tablespoons grated Gruyère cheese
¼ cup panko bread crumbs
1 teaspoon celery salt
½ teaspoon garlic powder

1½ tablespoons unsalted butter
1½ tablespoons all-purpose flour
2½ cups milk (2% is best here, but any will work)
¼ teaspoon celery salt
⅛ teaspoon freshly ground black pepper
2 cooked chicken breasts (see page 132), cubed
2 (12-ounce) bags mixed frozen vegetables

1. Preheat the oven to 375°F.

2. Bring a large pot of water to a boil. Add the pasta and cook until al dente according to the package directions. Drain and set aside in a 9 × 13-inch casserole dish.

3. In a small bowl, mix together all the topping ingredients. Set aside.

4. In the same pot that was used for the pasta, melt the butter over medium-low heat. Add the flour to the butter and whisk together with a wooden spoon for about 5 minutes until you have a lightly browned paste (this is a roux).

5. Add 1 cup of the milk and whisk well, breaking up any lumps. Stir in the remaining 1½ cups milk and increase the heat to medium-high. Cook, stirring often and occasionally scraping the bottom of the pan with the spoon, until the mixture has thickened and coats the spoon with little to no transparency, about 20 minutes. Add the celery salt and pepper and turn off the heat.

6. Stir in the pasta, chicken, and vegetables and mix until everything is covered in sauce. Transfer back to the casserole dish and sprinkle on the topping mixture. Bake for 15 minutes, or until the topping is crispy and the cheese is melted. Scoop it into bowls and serve.

What to Eat When You Go Out to Eat

So . . . you've got your healthy eating habits down at home, but what happens when you go out to a restaurant? This is where many people give up and quit their diets. Eating out is a big part of our culture, so not going out is not a reasonable option. We shouldn't feel as if we can't go out with friends and have something delicious at our favorite restaurant. . . . So how can you plan ahead so that your detox isn't derailed? What should you eat, what should you drink? What happens when you go overboard? How can you prepare yourself so you feel confident and comfortable ordering out?

Tips for Eating Out on a Calorie Budget

1. PLANNING IS KEY! Before you go out, look up the menu online. Look for healthy options and even call the restaurant to ask if they have any low-calorie dishes. Remember, you want to look for a dish that is veggie heavy, without too many carbs, and includes a lean protein. Still not sure? Pick a couple options and ask the waiter what he recommends.

2. SPLIT IT. What if you're going to your favorite burger place, or you simply can't leave the sports bar without enjoying your favorite nachos? Don't deprive yourself—share it with someone and enjoy it!

3. FILL UP ON WATER. As soon as you sit down, drink the water your waiter brings you and ask for more. The more water you drink, the fuller you'll be, and the less likely you'll be to overeat. Keep drinking that H_2O through your meal—it raises your metabolism!

4. DRINK SMART! In a perfect world, you won't be drinking alcohol if you're participating in one of the detox plans outlined in this book . . . but this world isn't perfect, and if you're going to splurge on a cocktail, we need to talk about what to order. Skip the sugary drinks, beer (I know, it sucks, I'm sorry), and the second and third round. More on the next page on what boozy drinks are smartest and what drinks will make you feel like you're splurging without all the calories and sugar.

5. WATCH OUT FOR FREEBIES! That bread that comes to the table, the tortilla chips—they're weight-loss Kryptonite. Ask your server to take it away! Now, if you went to the restaurant because they have the world's best rolls (*cough* Texas Roadhouse) or the

best chips and salsa in town, then (and only then) have some. Get a small plate and add half a roll or 10 chips, and nibble slowly on these treats so they don't run out before your meal comes. Oh, and go ahead and have all the salsa your little heart desires!

What to Drink

- SODA WATER. If a restaurant has a soda fountain, they probably have that little "soda" tab and will give you unlimited soda water. Ask for some lemon and lime wedges and squeeze those little metabolism-boosting jewels into your glass.
- HOT TEA AND ICED TEA (NOT SWEET TEA!). Zero calories and a little jolt of caffeine, yes, please! If you usually order a Rob Roy, ask for some lemon wedges for your iced tea. Skip the packets of fake sugar; if you absolutely must sweeten your drink, try a bit of honey or raw sugar.
- WINE AND COCKTAILS. Skip the sugary mixed drinks and order a glass of wine! At about 120 calories per glass, you can splurge and not blow your calorie budget. Other low-cal options are a martini at just 135 calories or a vodka soda (my personal favorite) at just 95 calories.

What to Eat

Of course we all know a salad is a great option when eating out, and should you find yourself at a restaurant with a salad you want to order, by all means go for it. But what if you're just salad-ed out? Here are some healthy meal ideas:

- REMEMBER YOUR PLATE EQUATION. Ideally you want your plate to contain more than 50 percent veggies, little to no refined carbs, and some lean protein. Think of the 50/25/25 equation in my first cookbook, *Lose Weight by Eating*: Look for a meal that is 50 percent (or more) veggies with some lean protein.
- LOOK FOR SMART SWAPS. At a burger place and see they have a turkey burger? Order that! Skip the mayo and get mustard and ketchup instead. What about a curry dish where you get to choose tofu or beef? You guessed it—choose the tofu, babe! Look for those smart swaps and you'll be looking smart in those tight jeans!
- WHEN IN DOUBT, CHICKEN! Just about every restaurant out there has a low-calorie chicken dish. Look for the words *grilled* or *rotisserie* and steer clear of fried and cheese- and cream-heavy chicken dishes.

- OPT FOR SMART SIDES. If fries, mashed potatoes, chips, or a fried side dish come with the meal, ask for a side salad or coleslaw, or simply ask them not to bring the side dish. Listen, I love potatoes (look in the index and you'll see how much), but restaurants tend to fry the heck out of them, and when they're not fried they're soaking in cream. Save your potato dishes for at home.

- RETHINK THAT APPETIZER. Do you really need it? If you're going out just for appetizer and a glass of wine, that's one thing, but if you're going out for a big meal, you don't also need an appetizer to start! You'll save both money and calories by skipping the apps, so do it!

- GET YOUR JUST DESSERT. I love my sweets, too, and I don't want to tell you that you can't have them. So let's talk about what to order and how to burn it off (*wink*). First, look for the fruit-heavy dessert. Next, you have to split it with someone, or you'll consume *way* too many empty calories. And finally, work it off, babe! Go dancing, take a walk . . . or (*hint hint*) take that dessert home and enjoy it, then work it off, in bed with your other half.

Help! I Went Overboard!

We all do it, and chances are I've gone overboard several times since I first typed these words. Life is short, so eat the chocolate, right?

You can't beat yourself up about this—you are human! Diets are hard to follow and you *will* fall off the wagon. It's what happens *after* you fall off that counts most, not the three slices of chocolate cake you ate! So, here's what you do:

1. GET OVER IT!
2. DON'T TRY TO SKIP A MEAL TO MAKE UP FOR IT. GET OVER IT!
3. DON'T SAY "I'LL START AGAIN TOMORROW." START AGAIN *NOW*. AND GET OVER IT!
4. DRINK A BIG GLASS OF WATER, PLAN YOUR NEXT HEALTHY MEAL, AND—YOU GUESSED IT—*GET OVER IT!*
5. YOU'RE HUMAN, AND YOU WILL MAKE MISTAKES, SO JUST EAT THE DAMN CHOCOLATE AND CUT YOURSELF SOME SLACK!

12

Breakfast and Brunch Detox Meals

We don't always have the time to putter around the kitchen in the morning, so in this chapter I pulled together fast, crave-worthy breakfasts that you can make during even the most hectic mornings, and some you can make ahead for even harder mornings.

Eating a well-rounded breakfast will keep you full for hours, and it helps you start the day off right so that you can make healthy choices all day long. So take the time to eat healthy in the a.m. . . . even if you have to eat standing up in the bathroom while drying your hair. (I've done it and recommend the English Muffin Sandwiches with Homemade Sausage Patties—you can enjoy them one-handed!)

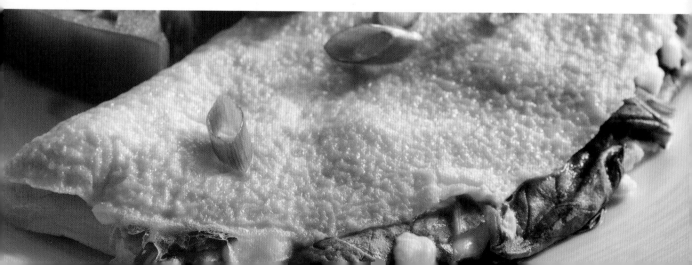

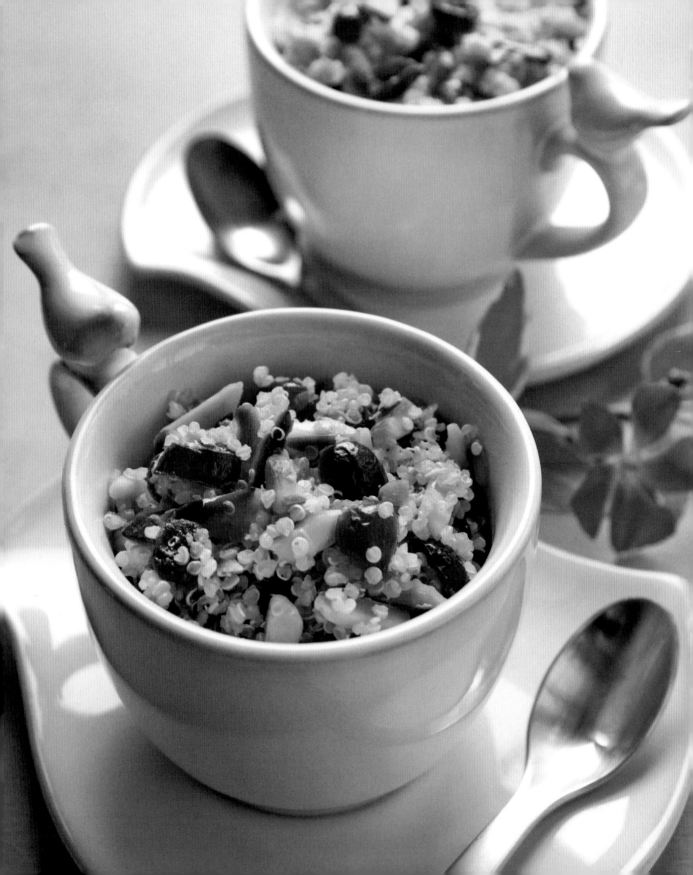

Lemon Cranberry Breakfast Quinoa

This is a great option for people who find oatmeal too mushy; quinoa has a firmer consistency. I find the nuts complement the quinoa and give more crunch to the meal, the lemon zest gives a boost of zero-calorie flavor, and, best of all, the cranberries plump up as you cook them.

You cook this undisturbed, which means you can get up, start breakfast, and jump in the shower. By the time you're out, your breakfast will be ready.

Makes 2 servings | Serving size: about ⅓ cup | Per serving: calories 296; fat 10 g; saturated fat 1 g; fiber 5 g; protein 9 g; carbohydrates 42.5 g; sugar 8.5 g | Prep time: 2 minutes | Cook time: 20 minutes

½ cup uncooked quinoa
2 teaspoons pure vanilla extract
Zest of 1 lemon
2 tablespoons dried cranberries
2 tablespoons slivered almonds
Pure maple syrup (optional)

1. Rinse the quinoa in cold water. In a small saucepan, combine the quinoa, vanilla, lemon zest, cranberries, and 1¼ cups water. Cover and bring to a simmer over medium heat, then turn the heat to the lowest setting and cook, undisturbed, until all the water is absorbed, about 20 minutes.

2. While the quinoa simmers away, toast the almonds in a dry pan over medium-low heat until they start to brown, stirring often, 3 to 5 minutes. Transfer them to a plate to cool.

3. Serve the quinoa in two bowls, topped with the almonds and a maple syrup drizzle, if desired, for your pickier eaters.

Coconut Banana Parfaits with Coconut Granola

If you haven't heard it yet, now you're hearing it from me—macadamia nuts are coming up in the superfood world. Packed with vitamin E, they add tons of moisture to your skin while giving you a youthful glow, and they also curb your appetite . . . bonus!

I like to make this for fast weekday breakfasts. I bake the granola ahead of time and store it in the pantry. On busy mornings, I can whip up these parfaits in less than 5 minutes! The granola is also great in the Açaí Bowl with Coconut Granola (page 47), and grown-ups and kids love it as a cereal—it's fantastic with coconut milk.

Makes 6 servings | Serving size: 1 parfait | Per serving: calories 336; fat 17 g; saturated fat 13.5 g; fiber 16 g; protein 12 g; carbohydrates 46 g; sugar 17 g
Prep time: 5 minutes | Cook time: 18 minutes (you can make it head of time!)

GRANOLA
2 cups old-fashioned rolled oats
¼ cup unsweetened coconut flakes
2 tablespoons coconut oil
2 tablespoons coconut sugar
2 tablespoons chopped macadamia nuts
2 tablespoons raw sunflower seeds
½ cup unsweetened applesauce

PARFAIT
3 small bananas (or 2 large), sliced into ¼-inch-thick rings
2 cups coconut yogurt or vanilla 0% Greek yogurt

1. Make the granola: Preheat the oven to 350°F.

2. In a 9 × 9-inch casserole dish, combine all the granola ingredients and mix well. Bake for 15 to 18 minutes, stirring twice, until golden brown. Leave uncovered on the countertop overnight to crisp up (or serve right away, but it will get crisper if it sits out).

3. Make the parfaits: In six clear glasses or mason jars, layer ¼ cup bananas, ⅓ cup yogurt, and ¼ cup coconut granola. Store leftover granola in an airtight container in your pantry for up to 2 weeks.

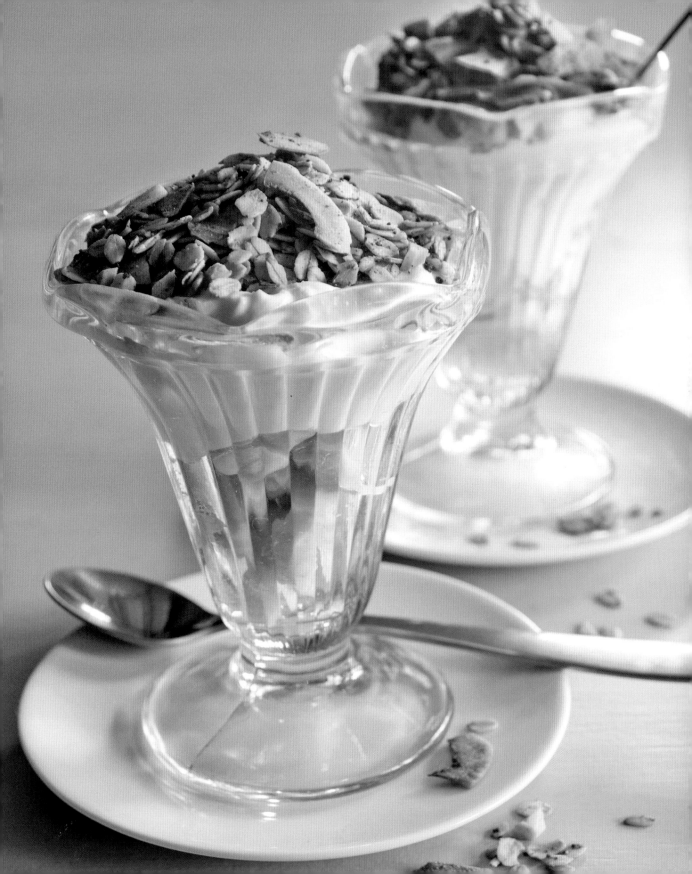

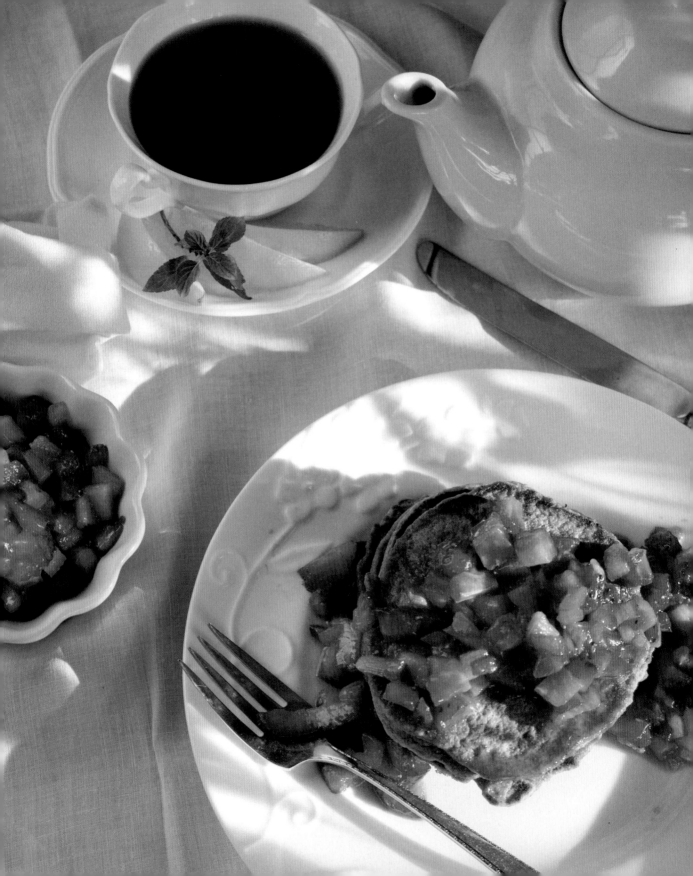

Strawberry Pancakes

Pink pancakes! That will get you out of bed in the morning.

I love the ease of these pancakes—you make the batter in a blender, saving lots of time. What I love most, though, is that you can then pour from the blender straight onto the griddle . . . even easier! And best of all, there's just a blender and a griddle to clean—no bowls and whisk—saving you time on cleanup as well as cooking.

Makes 2 servings | Serving size: 4 pancakes and ¼ cup strawberry topping
Per serving: calories 382; fat 2.5 g; saturated fat 0 g; fiber 10 g; protein 10 g;
carbohydrates 85 g; sugar 30 g | Prep time: 20 minutes | Cook time: 25 minutes

10 medium strawberries, hulled
⅓ cup almond or coconut milk
1 teaspoon pure vanilla extract
3 tablespoons pure maple syrup
1 cup whole wheat flour
1 teaspoon baking powder
Olive oil spray

STRAWBERRY TOPPING
10 medium strawberries
2 tablespoons powdered sugar

1. Place the strawberries, almond milk, vanilla, and maple syrup in a blender and blend until smooth.

2. Add the flour and baking powder and pulse until just combined; don't overblend or the pancakes will be tough. Let the batter rest for 15 minutes; it will fluff up a little. (You can even do this the night before and leave the batter in the fridge!)

3. Place a baking sheet in the oven. Preheat the oven to 200°F and preheat a griddle to medium heat.

4. Spray the griddle with oil spray and pour ¼-cup dollops of the batter onto the hot griddle. When the pancakes start bubbling all over (not just the edges), about 3 minutes, gently flip and cook the other side for 1 to 2 minutes, until lightly browned on the bottom.

5. As the pancakes are done, transfer them to the baking sheet in the oven to keep warm. Repeat to make the rest of the pancakes.

6. While the pancakes cook, hull and chop the strawberries. Place them in a small bowl, add the powdered sugar, and toss to coat the strawberries (you can also do this the night before and place in the fridge).

7. Serve the pancakes topped with the strawberries. Store leftover pancakes in a freezer bag in the refrigerator for up to 4 days or in the freezer for up to 3 months. Reheat in a toaster or a 250°F oven.

California Avocado Toast

Living in California, I saw some interesting new health-food trends. Some were way too far-out for me, but others were so amazing that I'm proud to have lived in this healthy foodie haven, where I got to try them first. My latest favorite craze is toast, and fancy restaurants adorn toasted bread with numerous toppings and charge up to $12 for one slice! I've spent the money at these places to try them (so you don't have to), and here I've included my favorite fancy toast.

Here's the thing about this recipe—you have to get the best bread possible. There are very few ingredients here, so you need each one to count.

Makes 4 servings | Serving size: 1 toast | Per serving: calories 228; fat 12 g; saturated fat 4 g; fiber 13.5 g; protein 8 g; carbohydrates 21.5 g; sugar 1 g | Prep time: 5 minutes | Cook time: 10 minutes

4 slices whole wheat sourdough bread
1 garlic clove, halved
1 avocado, sliced
1 large tomato, cut into 8 slices
½ cup shredded sharp cheddar cheese
½ cup sprouts
Hot sauce (optional)

1. Toast the bread in the toaster or place it on a baking sheet and bake for 5 to 8 minutes on each side in a 350°F oven (this works well if you're making lots of servings).

2. Preheat the broiler.

3. When the bread is cool enough to handle, place the toast slices on a baking sheet and rub the tops with the garlic clove. Divide the avocado, tomato, and cheese among the slices. Place under the broiler for 2 to 4 minutes, until the cheese is melted, watching closely so it doesn't burn.

4. Immediately top each slice with sprouts (the melted cheese will help the sprouts stick and stay put). Slice in half and serve with hot sauce (if using).

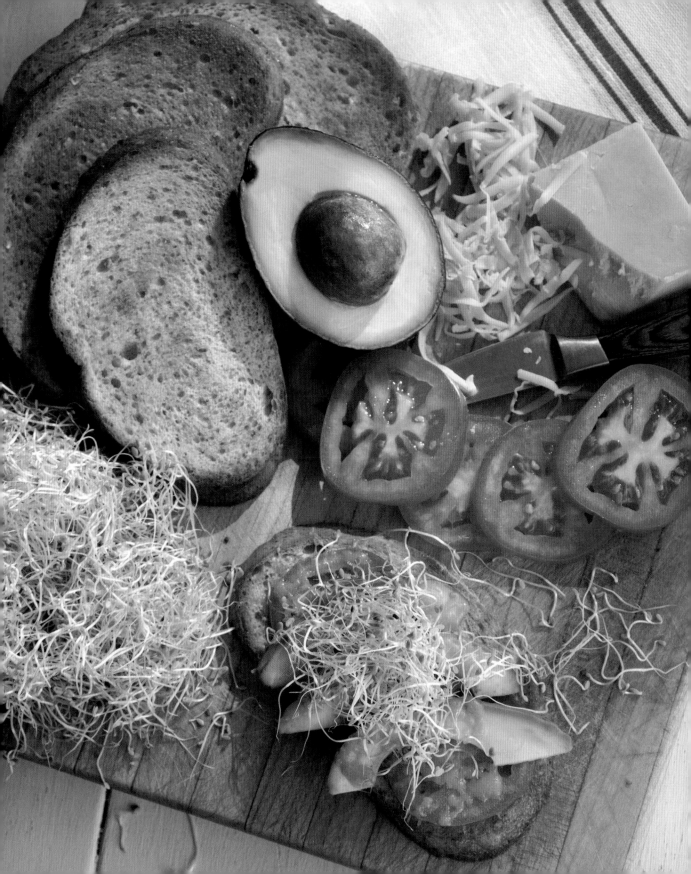

English Muffin Sandwiches with Homemade Sausage Patties

Skip that drive-thru! Save money and time and make it yourself! I make all six servings, wrap them individually in parchment paper, and stack them in a freezer bag for fast breakfasts.

I like to make my own sausage patties, but sometimes I use turkey bacon or skip the meat altogether. I've included variations below so you'll have lots of breakfast sandwich options.

Makes 6 servings | Serving size: 1 sandwich | Per serving: calories 350; fat 15 g; saturated fat 5 g; fiber 3 g; protein 28 g; carbohydrates 23 g; sugar 2 g | Prep time: 10 minutes | Cook time: 15 minutes

HOMEMADE SAUSAGE PATTIES
1 pound ground turkey
1 garlic clove, grated
8 fresh sage leaves, finely minced
½ teaspoon lemon zest
½ teaspoon ground cumin
½ teaspoon chili powder
½ teaspoon kosher salt
¼ teaspoon freshly ground black pepper

SANDWICHES
Olive oil spray
6 whole wheat English muffins
6 large eggs
½ cup shredded sharp cheddar cheese

1. Make the patties: In a medium bowl, mix together all the sausage ingredients until just combined; don't overmix or you'll have tough sausages.

2. Line a plate with a paper towel. Spray a large skillet with oil spray and place it over medium-high heat. Form the sausage mixture into 6 flat discs, placing them in the skillet as you work. Cook them for 1 to 2 minutes on each side, pressing down a little to help them retain their flat shape. When browned completely and cooked through, transfer them to the prepared plate to drain.

3. Make the sandwiches: Preheat the oven to 350°F. Spray 6 cups of a 12-cup muffin pan with oil spray.

4. Cut the English muffins in half and lay them cut side up on a baking sheet. Crack an egg into each muffin pan cup (add a little water to the empty cups to avoid scorching the pan).

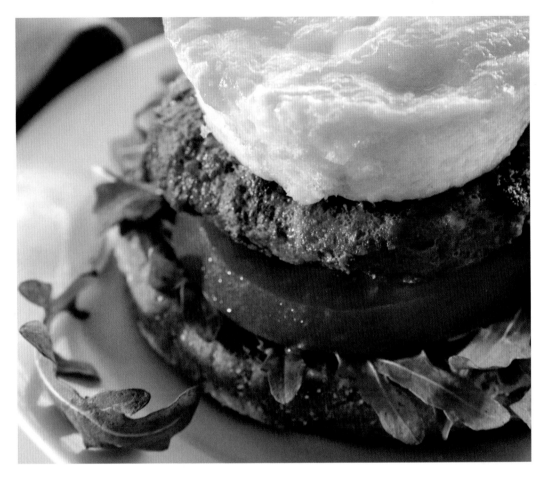

5. Place the English muffin sheet and the muffin pan in the oven and toast/bake for 5 minutes. Remove the English muffins, top each egg with 1½ tablespoons of the cheese, and bake for 5 more minutes, or until the cheese is melted and the eggs are firm.

6. Place a sausage patty on each English muffin bottom. Top with the egg and English muffin top. If you're making these ahead, wrap them in parchment paper and place them in a large freezer bag. Store in the refrigerator for up to 3 days or in the freezer for up to 3 months.

VARIATIONS

- Skip the sausage to make a vegetarian sandwich.
- Swap out the sausage for a slice of turkey bacon, cooked and halved.
- Add sliced tomato and arugula—my fave!

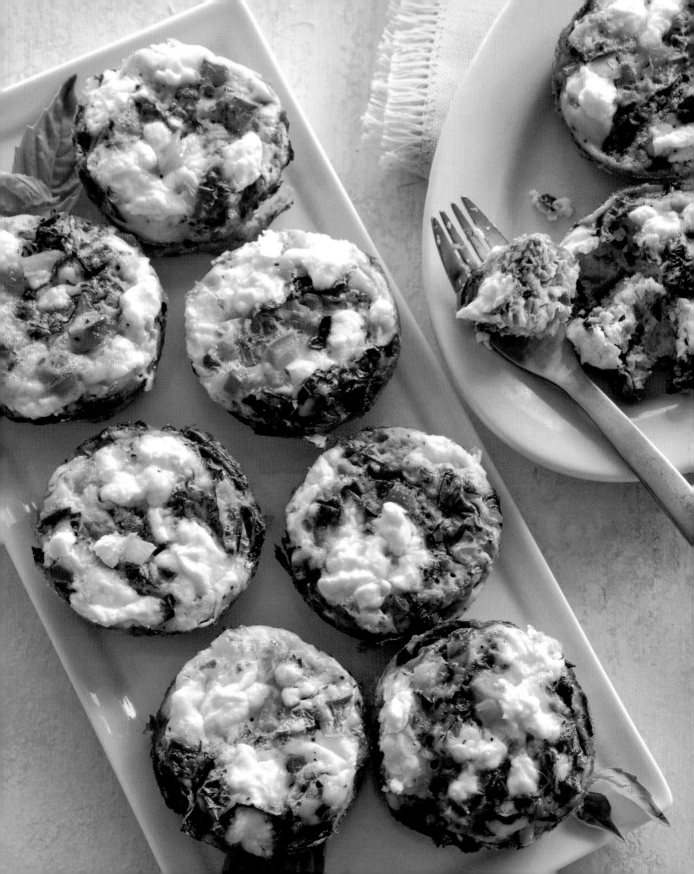

Muffin Cup Veggie Omelets

These easy omelets are great for breakfasts on the go. Wrap a couple in some parchment paper and enjoy on the road or at your desk; they can be eaten with your hands!

Save more time in the morning by prepping the omelets the night before. Fill the muffin cups with veggies and whisk the eggs in a bowl, cover both with plastic wrap, and place in the fridge. The next morning, give the eggs another quick whisk, then pour them into the muffin cups, top with cheese, and pop in the oven. This will take less than 5 minutes.

And finally, yes, you can reheat these for the very busiest mornings. Make and refrigerate them a few days ahead and pop them in a 200°F oven while you get ready. They need 20 minutes to heat, but can be left in the oven to stay warm for up to an hour.

Makes 6 servings | Serving size: 2 omelets | Per serving: calories 89; fat 5 g; saturated fat 3 g; fiber 5 g; protein 10 g; carbohydrates 2 g; sugar 1 g | Prep time: 15 minutes | Cook time: 20 minutes

Olive oil spray
½ cup chopped red bell pepper
¼ cup chopped onion
½ cup chopped white mushrooms
¼ cup chopped spinach
5 fresh basil leaves, chopped
4 large eggs
3 large egg whites
Pinch of kosher salt
Pinch of freshly ground black pepper
¼ cup crumbled goat cheese

1. Preheat the oven to 350°F. Spray a 12-cup muffin pan with oil spray.

2. As you chop the veggies, divide them among the muffin cups.

3. In a large bowl, whisk together the eggs, egg whites, salt, and pepper. Pour 2 tablespoons of the egg mixture into each muffin cup, then top each with 1 teaspoon of goat cheese.

4. Bake the omelets for 20 minutes, then let them rest for 5 minutes in the pan (this will help them stay together).

VARIATIONS

- You can use any cheese you like! Cheddar and feta both work well.
- If you like spice, add a few dashes of your favorite hot sauce to the eggs.
- If you want to add meat, crumble 2 cooked sausage patties (see page 220) and add them to the veggies.

Breakfast Tacos

Breakfast burritos are delicious, but breakfast tacos are something to be celebrated! Make them on (Taco) Tuesday mornings to get the kids out of bed and excited about their food, or any day of the week—kids love to eat with their hands!

Makes 10 servings | Serving size: 2 tacos | Per serving: calories 165; fat 6 g; saturated fat 1.5 g; fiber 3 g; protein 9 g; carbohydrates 19.5 g; sugar 3 g | Prep time: 5 minutes | Cook time: 15 minutes

Olive oil spray
1 medium onion, chopped
1 red bell pepper, chopped
1 garlic clove, chopped
1 jalapeño, ribs and seeds removed, chopped
¼ cup frozen corn
1 tablespoon chili powder
½ teaspoon ground cumin
1 tablespoon chopped fresh cilantro, or
   1 teaspoon dried
Pinch of kosher salt
Pinch of freshly ground black pepper
10 large eggs
20 (6-inch) corn tortillas

OPTIONAL TOPPINGS
Chopped fresh cilantro
Avocado slices
Grated sharp cheddar cheese
0% Greek yogurt
Hot sauce or salsa
Pickled jalapeño slices
Lime wedges

1. Spray a large skillet with oil spray and place over medium heat. Add the onion, bell pepper, garlic, jalapeño, corn, chili powder, cumin, and cilantro. Sprinkle with the salt and pepper and cook until the onion and bell pepper are soft, about 10 minutes.

2. In a large bowl, whisk together the eggs. Push all the veggies to one side of the skillet and pour the eggs on the other side. Scramble until almost set, then mix with the veggies. When the eggs are almost done cooking, remove them from the heat (they'll continue to cook).

3. Serve the eggs in the tortillas and offer the optional toppings. I love these with pickled jalapeños, extra cilantro, and a good squirt of lime juice.

If you're not going to make all 20 tacos at once, do as I do: Chop up the onion, bell pepper, garlic, and jalapeño and toss all of it into a gallon-size freezer bag. Add the corn, chili powder, cumin, cilantro, and a pinch each of salt and pepper, and shake it all up. Use ¼ cup of this mixture for each serving (so if you need 2 servings, scoop out ½ cup), then leave the ¼-cup measure in the bag for easy measurement later. Toss the entire bag into the freezer. For each serving, you'll need 1 egg and 2 tortillas.

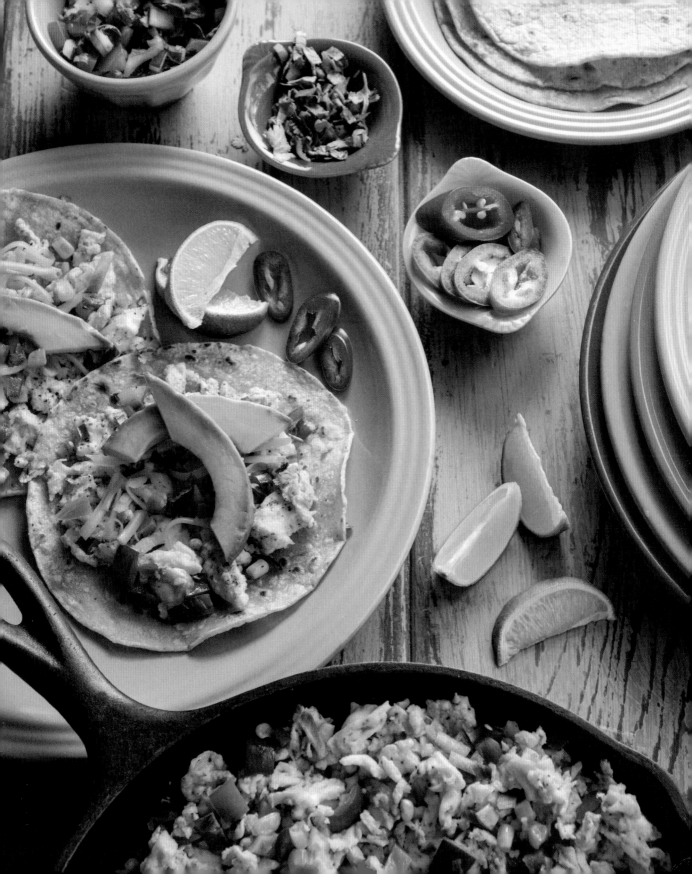

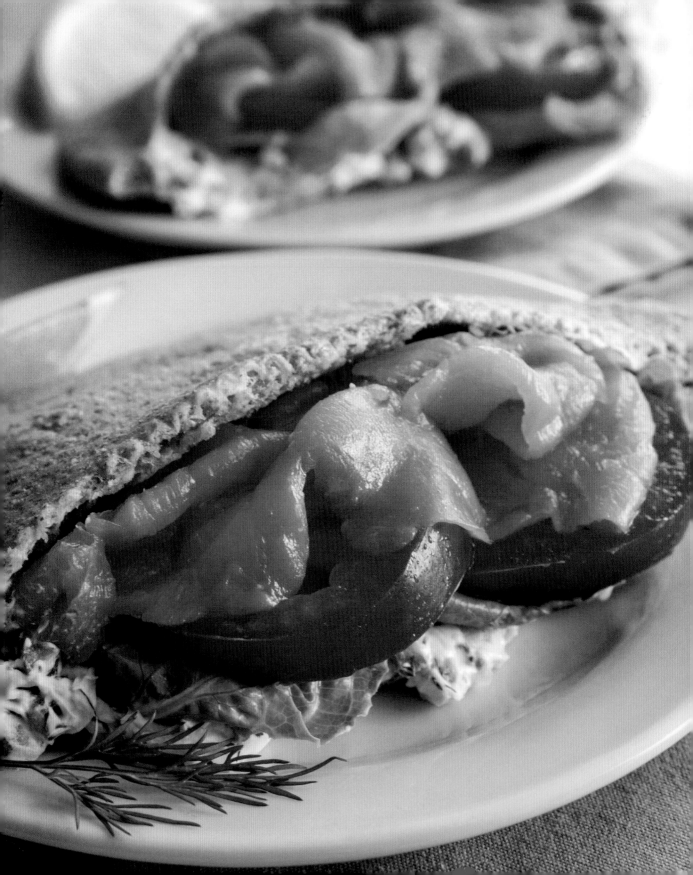

Smoked Salmon Breakfast Pita

So, yeah, this is in the breakfast chapter, but this salmon is fantastic for lunch and dinner, too! It also travels very well and makes a great brunch on the go.

Salmon is such a great breakfast protein; it's packed full of omega-3s and vitamin B_{12} for a healthy, beautiful body. This beauty food will make your hair and skin glow, plus, it's packed full of healthy fats. Healthy fats supply your body with the fat it craves, and by doing so tells your body to release excess fat it's "storing" for times of low-fat eating. This will help your body reduce fat faster!

Makes 2 servings | Serving size: 1 pita | Per serving: calories 166; fat 5 g; saturated fat 2 g; fiber 3 g; protein 12 g; carbohydrates 19 g; sugar 1.5 g | Prep time: 5 minutes | Cook time: 0 minutes

3 tablespoons low-fat cream cheese
1 tablespoon chopped fresh dill
1 tablespoon chopped red onion
1 tablespoon capers, drained, rinsed, and chopped
2 whole wheat pitas
2 romaine leaves, halved
1 small tomato, cut into ½-inch-thick slices
4 smoked salmon slices
Lemon wedges (optional)

1. In a small bowl, smash together the cream cheese, dill, onion, and capers with the back of a fork until combined.

2. Halve the pitas and gently open them up. Smear the bottom halves with the cream cheese mixture and top with romaine, tomato slices, and smoked salmon. Serve with lemon wedges (if using) to squeeze over the filling.

Cranberry Oatmeal Muffins

Ohhh, you're gonna love these! Not only are they filling, but you can also make them in a blender, making them super easy!

One very important note: Whenever you blend oatmeal, washing or at least soaking your blender right away is paramount, or you'll have oatmeal cement in your blender. Do as I do: As soon as you pour the last muffin, move the blender to the sink and add hot water and soap right away. When you have the muffins doing their thing in the oven, you can clean out your blender with ease.

Makes 12 servings | Serving size: 1 muffin | Per serving: calories 118; fat 2 g; saturated fat 5 g; fiber 2 g; protein 3 g; carbohydrates 22.5 g; sugar 10 g | Prep time: 10 minutes | Cook time: 20 minutes

Olive oil spray
1 banana
1 cup almond or coconut milk
1 large egg
2 tablespoons honey
Zest of 1 lemon
2½ cups old-fashioned rolled oats
2 teaspoons baking powder
½ teaspoon baking soda
½ cup dried cranberries

1. Preheat the oven to 350°F. Spray a 12-cup muffin pan with oil spray.

2. Place the banana, almond milk, egg, and honey in a blender and blend until smooth. Add the lemon zest, oats, baking powder, and baking soda and blend until smooth. Fold in the cranberries. That was easy!

3. Use an ice cream scoop to fill the prepared muffin cups two-thirds full. Bake for 20 minutes, then let the muffins cool in the pan for 10 minutes before popping them out and serving. Watch out for muffin thieves—little children love to steal these!

Southwestern Tofu Scramble

I am not a fan of tofu. There, I said it! But I could eat this dish every single day. Packed with veggies and topped with my favorite hot sauce, it's heavenly! Give it a try, and if you really can't stand the tofu, swap it out for 1 cup egg whites and make a more traditional scramble.

Makes 4 servings | Serving size: about 1½ cups | Per serving: calories 144; fat 10.5 g; saturated fat 1 g; fiber 2 g; protein 13 g; carbohydrates 9 g; sugar 2.5 g
Prep time: 15 minutes | Cook time: 20 minutes

16 ounces extra-firm tofu
1 teaspoon chili powder
1 teaspoon garlic powder
⅛ teaspoon kosher salt
⅛ teaspoon freshly ground black pepper
Olive oil spray
1 red bell pepper, chopped
1 jalapeño, ribs and seeds removed, chopped
½ red onion, chopped
2 cups kale, stems removed, leaves thinly sliced
Chopped fresh cilantro (optional)
Hot sauce (optional)

1. Wrap the tofu in a clean tea towel and place it under a heavy object, such as a cast-iron skillet, for 15 minutes to draw out some of the moisture.

2. Meanwhile, in a small bowl, mix together the chili powder, garlic powder, salt, pepper, and 2 tablespoons water. Set aside.

3. Lightly spray a large sauté pan with oil spray and place it over medium heat. Add the bell pepper, jalapeño, and onion and cook, stirring occasionally, until the veggies are soft, about 10 minutes.

4. Add the kale, turn the heat to low, and cover the pan. Cook for about 2 minutes, until the kale starts to wilt. Scoot all the veggies to one side of the pan.

5. Unwrap the tofu and use a fork to crumble it. Place it in the sauté pan and cook for 3 minutes. Pour the chili powder mixture over the tofu, and stir to combine. Cook for about 2 minutes more, until the chili powder mixture is absorbed, then serve topped with cilantro and your favorite hot sauce (if using).

Feta and Spinach Omelet

So easy, so delicious! Don't you agree that sometimes the simplest recipes can be the yummiest? Make sure to get good-quality ingredients, as each one is carrying a lot of weight in this recipe.

I like to get a block of feta as opposed to precrumbled feta; it's easier to use in recipes like the Greek Salad Skewers on page 282, and I find that a block lasts longer in the fridge.

Makes 1 serving | Serving size: 1 omelet | Per serving: calories 165; fat 11.5 g; saturated fat 3.5 g; fiber 0.5 g; protein 13 g; carbohydrates 1.5 g; sugar 0.5 g | Prep time: 2 minutes | Cook time: 5 minutes

Olive oil spray
2 large eggs
1 tablespoon crumbled feta cheese
Heaping ¼ cup baby spinach
1 green onion, thinly sliced

1. Lightly spray a small skillet with oil and place over medium heat.

2. In a medium bowl, whisk together the eggs with ½ teaspoon water. Pour the eggs into the hot skillet and cook, undisturbed, until they start to bubble up and pull away from the sides of the pan.

3. Add half the cheese on one side of the omelet, top with spinach (it looks like a lot, but it will wilt down), and top with the remaining cheese. Fold the bare side of the omelet over the side with the spinach and cheese and cook for 2 minutes. Flip and cook for 2 minutes more.

4. Transfer the omelet to a plate and top with the green onion.

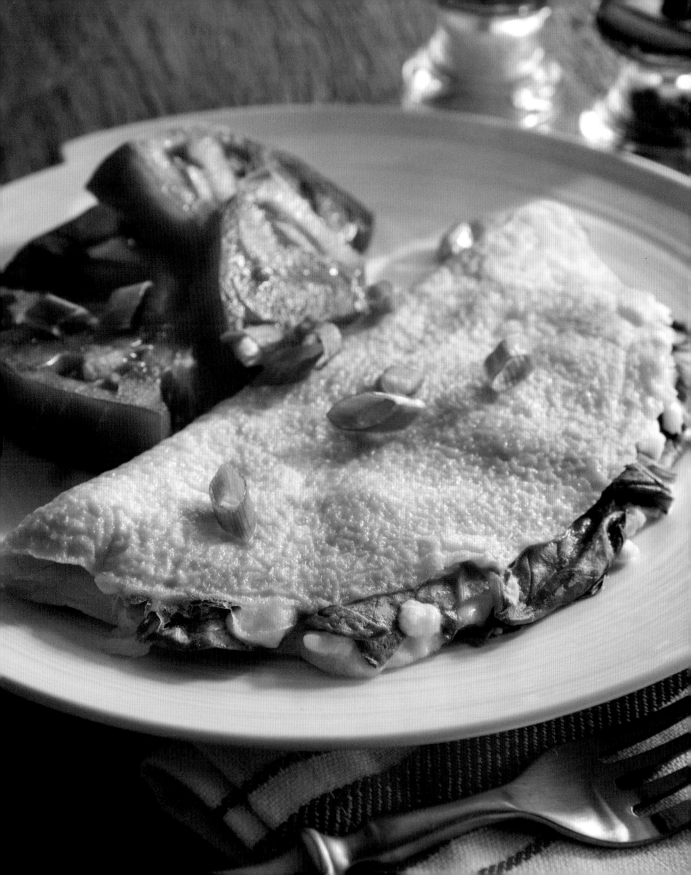

13

Detox Drinks and Mocktails

Sorry, friends, no booze in this book. It's a detox book, after all. But if you're wondering what counts as a healthy alcohol drink while on these plans, my answer is always *wine*, in small amounts! Wine is loaded with antioxidants, it's good for your heart, and it's all natural.

I've included lots of natural soda options for those of you looking to kick the sugary soda habit, water drinks to help you get in your gallon every day and actually enjoy it, and of course some coffeehouse copycats to save you money and hundreds of calories.

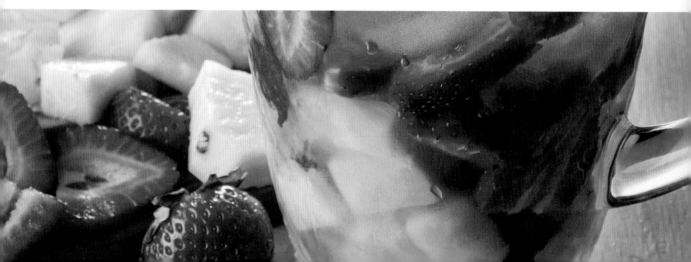

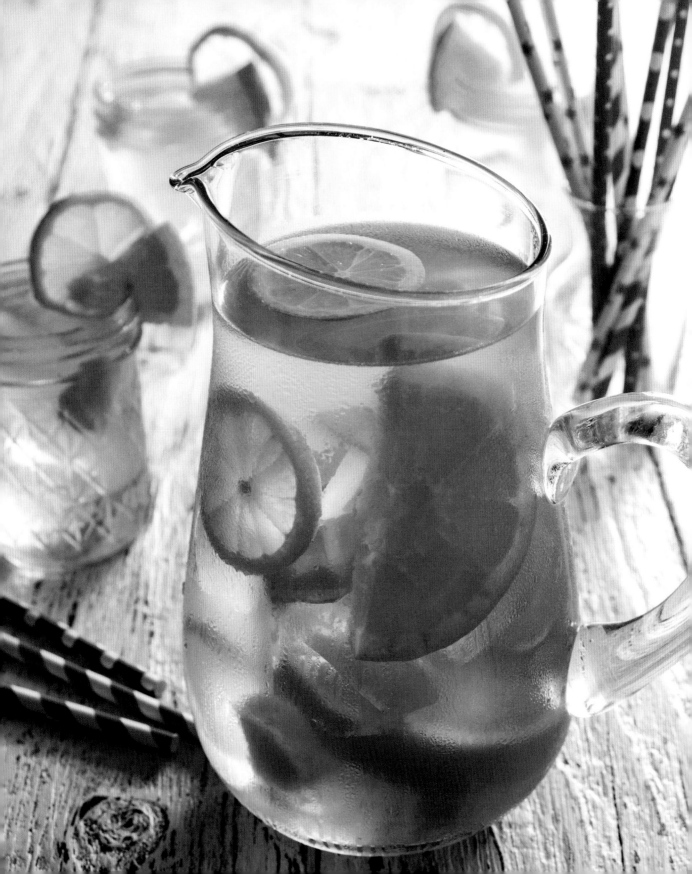

"Hey There, Hot Stuff" Infused Green Iced Tea

Hey there, beautiful, here's a drink that will boost your metabolism and make you glow! The green tea naturally raises your metabolism, as do the lemon, orange, ginger, and pineapple!

The high concentration of vitamin C in this drink will help give you a youthful glow, clear up your skin, and reduce redness and dullness on your face. So drink up and feel beautiful, hot stuff!

Makes 8 servings | Serving size: 1 cup | Per serving: calories 4; fat 0 g; saturated fat 0 g; fiber 0 g; protein 0 g; carbohydrates 1 g; sugar 1 g | Prep time: 5 minutes | Infuse time: 15 minutes

¼ cup sliced peeled fresh ginger
5 organic green tea bags, with the paper tags cut off
1 lemon, thinly sliced
1 orange, thinly sliced
¼ cup fresh or frozen mango chunks
¼ cup fresh or frozen pineapple chunks

1. Pour 8 cups water into a medium saucepan, add the ginger, and bring to a boil over medium-high heat. Remove from the heat, add the tea bags, and steep for about 15 minutes. Strain the brewed tea into a glass pitcher and discard the ginger and tea bags. Add the lemon, orange, mango, and pineapple and let cool to room temperature, then refrigerate.

2. Serve over ice. The iced tea will keep in the refrigerator for 48 hours.

VARIATIONS

- Most people find the tea sweet enough with the mango and pineapple, but if you're looking for a sweeter tea, brew it with fresh or dried stevia leaves, or add raw honey in moderation while the tea is still hot.
- If you prefer hot tea, in a mug, pour hot water over a green tea bag and a thin slice of ginger. Steep for 5 minutes, then remove the tea bag and ginger and add a squeeze of lemon and an orange wedge. Toss in a chunk of room-temperature mango and pineapple and enjoy.

Cucumber, Lime, and Mint Water

Cucumbers are great for detoxing your body; they reduce bloat, swelling, and help your tummy look flatter. Limes naturally increase your metabolism, speeding up your weight loss and giving you a boost of vitamin C. The mint also helps to reduce bloat, so if you're feeling a little puffy, make a batch of this yummy drink and give your body a boost of bloat-reducing goodness.

I never make this drink the same way twice! You'll find some optional add-ins in the ingredients, so you, too, can get creative and find your favorite combinations.

Makes 4 servings | Serving size: 2 cups | Per serving: calories 0; fat 0 g saturated fat 0 g; fiber 0 g; protein 0 g; carbohydrates 0 g; sugar 0 g | Prep time: 3 minutes | Infuse time: 2 to 24 hours

1 lime, sliced into thin rings
1 small cucumber, sliced into thin rings

OPTIONAL ADD-INS
1 lemon, thinly sliced
½ cup diced fresh or frozen pineapple (for a tropical sweet twist)
½ cup sliced fresh or frozen strawberries (for even more metabolism-boosting vitamin C)

1. Add the limes, cucumber, and any of the add-ins to a large pitcher. Top with ice, which will hold down the ingredients, and fill the pitcher with water.

2. Let the water infuse for at least 2 hours or up to overnight in the fridge before serving. If you like your water at room temperature, let it infuse on the countertop, but be sure to add the ice to hold down the fruit (or use an infusion pitcher, which will hold the ingredients underwater without the ice).

Mango, Cucumber, and Basil Water

My dearly departed friend Tanya taught me how to make "spa waters." It all started back when I was in my early twenties, and more than fifteen years later, fruit-infused waters are still a huge part of my daily life. In the short amount of time that Tanya graced this world, she taught me more about what it means to be a woman, a good friend, and a mentor than words could ever express, and I celebrate that amazing woman here by sharing with you her very favorite drink.

We loved making this together as roommates, and whether she knew it or not, this was a very healthy drink! It helps reduce bloat, thanks to the cucumber and mint, and the mango raises metabolism, boosts memory, and even increases the libido. Tanya would get a laugh out of that!

Makes 4 servings | Serving size: 2 cups | Per serving: calories 5; fat 0 g; saturated fat 0 g; fiber 0 g; protein 0 g; carbohydrates 1 g; sugar 0.5 g | Prep time: 3 minutes | Infuse time: 2 to 24 hours

---

1 mango, peeled and cut into large chunks (reserve the pits)
1 small cucumber, thinly sliced
3 large or 5 small fresh basil leaves

1. Place the mango in a large pitcher. Squeeze the juice from the pit into the pitcher and drop it in as well. Add the cucumber and twist the basil leaves as you drop them into the pitcher to bruise them and release their flavor. Top with ice, which will hold down the ingredients, and fill the pitcher with water.

2. Let the water infuse for at least 2 hours or up to overnight in the fridge before serving. If you like your water at room temperature, let it infuse on the countertop, but be sure to add the ice to hold down the fruit (or use an infusion pitcher, which will hold the ingredients underwater without the ice).

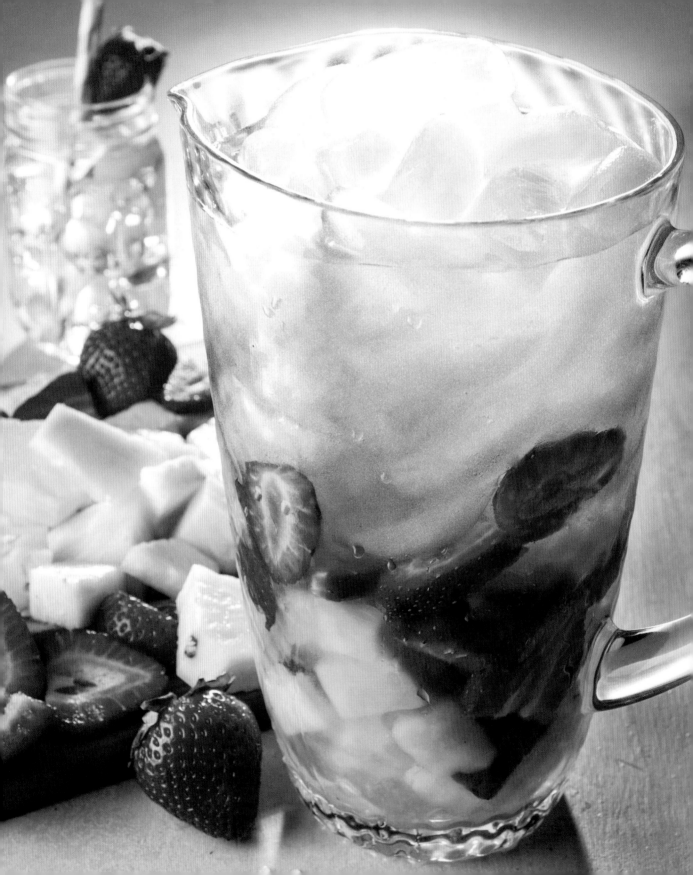

Pineapple Strawberry Infused Water

This one goes out to all you sweet-toothed readers out there. If you're trying to stop drinking sugar-packed juice or sodas, this refreshing water will make your day! It's packed full of flavor, so you can start drinking up and slimming down.

Both the strawberries and the pineapple naturally boost metabolism, so stop adding empty calories and put down that can of soda—pick up a glass of this yummy fruit-infused water instead!

Makes 4 servings | Serving size: 2 cups | Per serving: calories 6; fat 0 g; saturated fat 0 g; fiber 0 g; protein 0 g; carbohydrates 1 g; sugar 1 g | Prep time: 3 minutes | Infuse time: 2 to 24 hours

1 cup cubed fresh or frozen pineapple
8 fresh or frozen strawberries, hulled and quartered if fresh

1. Place the pineapple and strawberries in a large pitcher. Top with ice, which will hold down the ingredients, and fill the pitcher with water.

2. Let the water infuse for at least 2 hours or up to overnight in the fridge before serving. If you like your water at room temperature, let it infuse on the countertop, but be sure to add the ice to hold down the fruit (or use an infusion pitcher, which will hold the ingredients underwater without the ice).

Mojito-Flavored Soda

Soda . . . such a negative word in weight loss, and for good reason—diet sodas cause fat storage and weight gain, and sugar-packed sodas are full of empty calories that add weight to your midsection.

So what do you do if you have a fierce soda habit? Try one of my all-natural sodas, like this yummy mojito version. Packed full of metabolism-boosting and slimming ingredients, it will help you feel and look amazing, and best of all, the bubbles in this drink curb your soda cravings. So drink up and slim down!

*Makes 15 servings | Serving size: **8 ounces** | Per serving: **calories 0; fat 0 g; saturated fat 0 g; fiber 0 g; protein 0 g; carbohydrates 0 g; sugar 0 g** | Prep time: **5 minutes** | Infuse time: **2 to 4 hours***

2 (2-liter) bottles sparkling water
3 limes, thinly sliced
1 orange, thinly sliced
½ cup fresh mint leaves

1. Pour out about ⅓ cup of the sparkling water from both 2-liter bottles (I pour it into a glass and drink it while I work, yum!). This will make room for the fruit.

2. Add the limes, oranges, and mint leaves to the bottles, rolling the citrus slices as you work so they will fit. Close up tightly and place in the fridge to infuse for 2 to 4 hours before serving over ice.

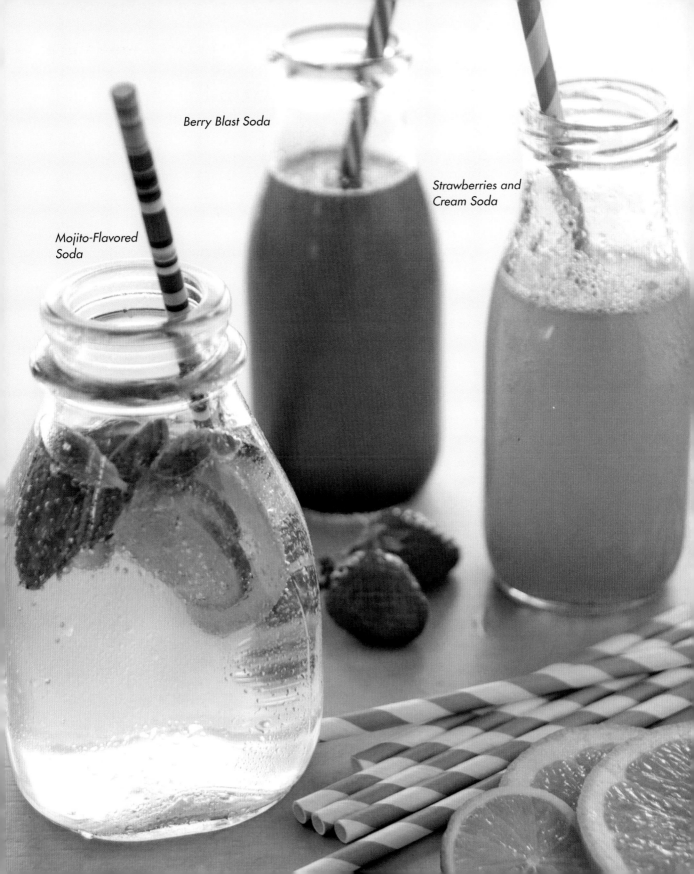

Berry Blast Soda

Strawberries and
Cream Soda

Mojito-Flavored
Soda

Strawberries and Cream Soda

Yummy, I love all things "strawberries and cream," as you well know if you have my first cookbook (strawberries and cream cookies, anyone?). I always loved those flavored cream sodas when I was a kid, and as it turns out, this is my daughter's favorite drink. (I'm so proud: She likes makeup, chocolate, and this soda—she is so *my* daughter!)

This soda is great for sipping all day long, to serve at parties, and even to pack in kids' lunch boxes. With just a single teaspoon of honey in eight servings, you can feel good about drinking it whenever you like. Local honey is beneficial if you're allergy-prone, so try to seek that out.

Makes 8 servings | Serving size: 8 ounces | Per serving: calories 11; fat 0 g; saturated fat 0 g; fiber 0.5 g; protein 0 g; carbohydrates 2.5 g; sugar 2 g | Prep time: 1 minute | Cook time: 1 minute

15 fresh or frozen strawberries, hulled if fresh
1 teaspoon pure vanilla extract
1 teaspoon honey
1 (2-liter) bottle club soda

1. Place the strawberries, vanilla, and honey in a blender, add 2 tablespoons water, and blend. If needed to get the blender going, add more water, but just 1 to 2 tablespoons at a time; it will be thick. Transfer the sauce to a mason jar for storage until ready to use. The sauce will get better as it sits and will keep for up to 1 week in the fridge.

2. To serve, pour 8 ounces club soda into a glass, add 2 tablespoons of the strawberry sauce, and stir. Do not premix all the strawberry sauce with all the club soda unless you're serving it right away, or the bubbles will go flat. If serving at a party, mix the strawberry sauce and club soda in a large pitcher and serve immediately over ice.

Photo on page 241.

Berry Blast Soda

This all-natural soda is easy, delicious, and actually good for you! Did you know that berries naturally boost your metabolism and promote a healthy heart?

Unlike a fruit-infused water, you can make this in a manner of minutes, so do yourself a favor and keep a bag of frozen berries in your freezer year-round. Any time you want to grab for a calorie- or chemical-packed soda, make this instead. You'll be happy to find this healthy drink will curb your cravings for the bad stuff.

Makes 8 servings | Serving size: 8 ounces | Per serving: calories 11; fat 0 g; saturated fat 0 g; fiber 0.5 g; protein 0 g; carbohydrates 3 g; sugar 2 g | Prep time: 1 minute | Cook time: 1 minute

1 cup frozen mixed berries
1 teaspoon honey
1 (2-liter) bottle club soda

1. Place the berries and honey in a blender, add ¼ cup water, and blend. If needed to get the blender going, add more water, but just 1 or 2 tablespoons at a time; it will be thick. Transfer the berry sauce to a mason jar for storage until ready to use. The sauce will get better as it sits and will keep for up to 1 week in the fridge.

2. To serve, pour 8 ounces club soda into a glass, add 2 tablespoons of the berry sauce, and stir. Do not premix all the berry sauce with all the club soda unless you're serving it right away, or the bubbles will go flat. If serving at a party, mix the berry sauce and club soda in a large pitcher and serve over ice immediately.

Photo on page 241.

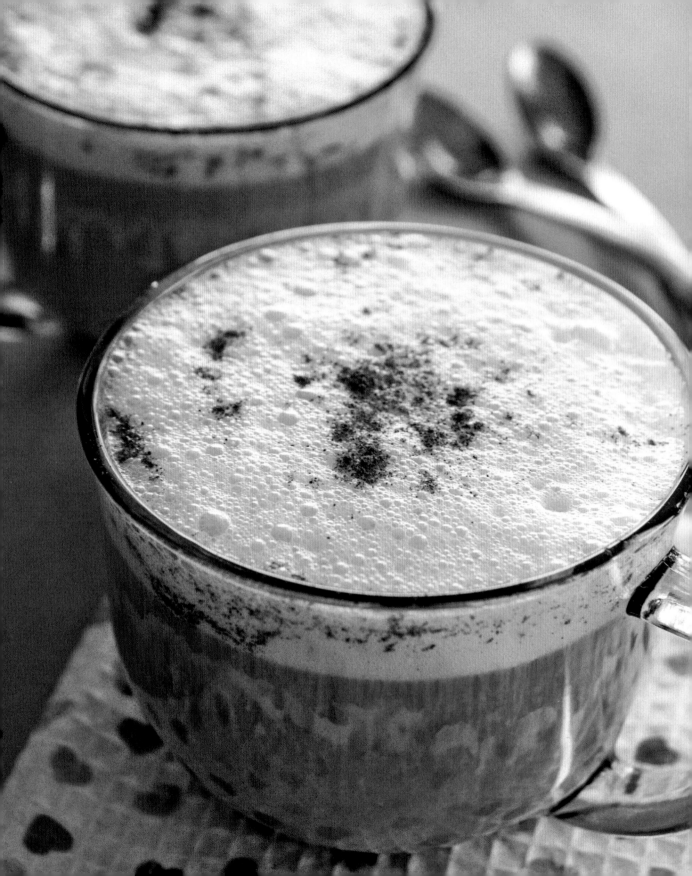

Skinny Chai Tea Latte

Oh, the irony . . . I'm typing this at a coffeehouse. I'm just trying to be honest here, because though I don't often visit coffeehouses, I do once in a while when I need a quiet space to work. I made this recipe earlier today, then figured, "What the heck, let's make sure it's as good as Starbucks," so I headed on over to my local spot and ordered—you guessed it—a chai tea latte. So here I am, drinking my second chai tea latte of the day and typing up my recipe, which I think tastes exactly the same.

I whisk the milk by hand, and it's very easy! It only takes a minute and you're done (and by the way, I've had two wrist surgeries in my whisking hand, so I assure you anyone can handle this mild activity).

Makes 2 servings | Serving size: 2 cups | Per serving: calories 112; fat 2.5 g; saturated fat 0 g; fiber 1 g; protein 1 g; carbohydrates 21 g; sugar 19 g | Prep time: 2 minutes | Cook time: 5 minutes

3 chai tea bags, with the paper tags cut off (I like Trader Joe's chai tea)
2 cups unsweetened almond milk
2 tablespoons pure maple syrup
Pumpkin pie spice (optional)

1. Heat 2 cups water to a simmer in a small saucepan, remove from the heat, and add the tea bags. Steep for 5 minutes.

2. Meanwhile, heat the almond milk in a small saucepan over medium-low heat. As soon as it's simmering, whisk it. Really get that whisk moving to create a thick foam.

3. Pour 1 cup of the tea into two large coffee or travel mugs and top with frothy milk and a sprinkle of pumpkin pie spice (if using). Congratulations, you just saved yourself $5.04.

Mexican Chocolate Latte

Go ahead and put on the movie *Chocolat....* I'll wait here. Honestly, do I really need to explain why this is so yummy? The look on Judi Dench's face when she drinks the chile-spiked hot chocolate should be enough to explain.

I made this skinny version with the help of my favorite beverage, coffee! If you follow me on Instagram, you already know I'm a coffee fanatic, but did you know that coffee naturally boosts metabolism, is packed with antioxidants, and can even lessen depression? In the case of this drink, I use zero-calorie coffee to dilute the chocolate, leaving you with a low-calorie version of the original decadent chocolate beverage ... or shall I say *Chocolat* beverage?

Makes 2 servings | Serving size: 1 cup | Per serving: calories 42; fat 1.5 g; saturated fat 0 g; fiber 1.5 g; protein 1 g; carbohydrates 7 g; sugar 5 g | Prep time: 1 minute | Cook time: 2 minutes

1 cup unsweetened almond milk
2 teaspoons unsweetened cocoa powder
¼ teaspoon chili powder
½ teaspoon ground cinnamon
½ teaspoon honey, plus more as needed to sweeten
1 cup hot strong-brewed coffee

1. In a small saucepan, heat the almond milk, cocoa powder, chili powder, cinnamon, and honey over medium-low heat until warmed to taste. Whisk briskly and continuously until foamy, 1 to 2 minutes.

2. Remove from the heat and stir in the coffee. Serve hot, or cool in the refrigerator for an hour and pour over ice for an iced chocolate latte.

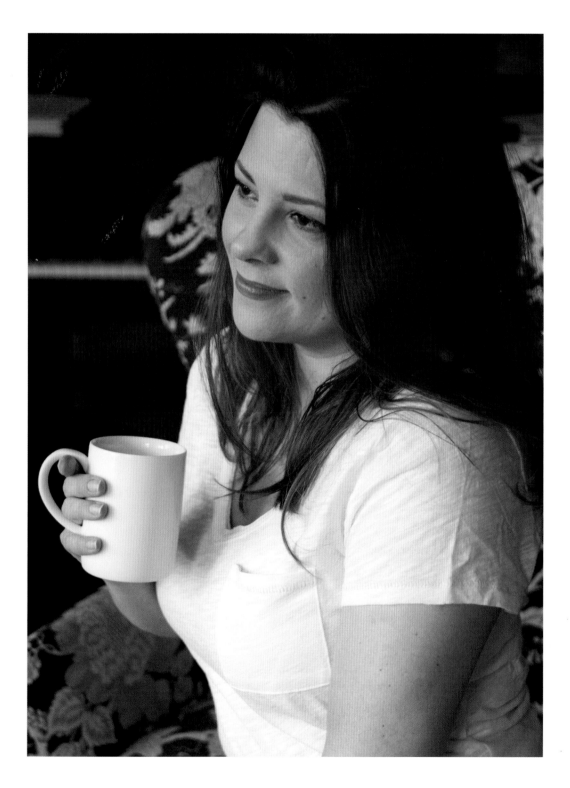

Tips for Keeping Coffee and Tea All Natural

You might be wondering why there's coffee in a book about detoxing. Well, if you'd read the introduction, and I'm totally offended if you haven't already (just kidding), you already know this book is "detox light," aka detox for everyone.

Years ago I tried to quit coffee. I was on a detox plan and was told that coffee was really bad for me and that I needed to quit. That lasted about a week before I had a complete coffee breakdown and quit the entire program . . . and it was an otherwise reasonable plan aside from the lack of caffeine. I don't want this to happen to you—I want you to find these plans reasonable and sustainable. I came to the conclusion that I was probably never gonna give up my love for coffee, and I'm okay with that. (I don't plan on giving up wine or chocolate either—but I digress.)

So while researching coffee for an article on my website, you'll never guess what I found out—coffee is actually good for you! It's packed full of antioxidants, boosts your metabolism, helps prevent diabetes and liver disease, protects against heart disease and stroke, and has a slew of other health benefits. So if you love coffee, just drink it and get over the stigma. Now, with that said, there are healthy and unhealthy ways to enjoy your cup of joe, so let's talk about that.

Coffee and Tea

Organic is best! Have you heard the news? Tea companies don't always wash the herbs before drying them. So yep, there's a good chance that all those pesticides are in your tea. And how do those chemicals taste? (Yuck!) In the case of coffee, they do wash the beans, but they've still been grown in pesticides—not good for your body! Choose organic whenever possible (Trader Joe's and Amazon have great low-price options).

Creamer

Have you used those fancy seasonal creamers? Of course you have—we all have. What you may not know is that they are packed full of chemicals, artificial sweeteners, and synthetic flavoring and will hinder your weight-loss and detox efforts. I gave them up years ago and I can't stand them anymore. Now that I go all natural with my beverages, I can taste and smell the chemicals in most store-bought creamers, and I'm completely grossed out by the strange film they leave on coffee cups (what do you think that does to your teeth and body?).

Here are my favorite healthy creamer options:

- COCONUT CREAMER: Trader Joe's has its own brand that's just like half-and-half. I love it, and it lasts forever in the fridge!

- ALMOND MILK CREAMER: My food stylist turned me onto Califia almond milk creamer. It's fantastic, sweet (no need for sugar), and all natural. There are many options out there; just be sure to read the ingredients—you want a short list of all-natural ingredients.

- NATURAL BLISS: You may want to sit down. So I just bagged on Coffeemate, and here I am telling you it's okay? Well, Coffeemate Natural Bliss has a great all-natural line of dairy and nondairy creamers. They can be a little pricey, but because they're sweet, you won't need the fancy organic sugar I'm about to talk about. Perfect for those of you who love traditional store-bought creamers.

- ORGANIC HALF-AND-HALF: If you're not looking to lose weight but just want to be healthier, try an organic half-and-half with one of the sugar options below.

Here are my healthy sweetener options:

- COCONUT SUGAR is lower on the glycemic index than sugar, and the manufacturing process is more natural than that of traditional sugar. It's a better option yet still high in calories, so use in moderation.

- STEVIA IN THE RAW: I am not a huge fan of zero-calorie sweeteners, however natural they are. For most people, a low-calorie count translates to "I can have as much as I like," and that's dangerous! Even low-calorie sweeteners will make you crave more sweet foods and carbohydrates. Sure, Stevia in the Raw is a good, healthy option, but don't go crazy with it, as it will still trigger you to crave more unhealthy foods. Remember: moderation!

- HONEY AND PURE MAPLE SYRUP: I love adding both to my coffee, and honey is already used often in tea. Both are healthy all-natural options. I specifically love maple syrup in my coffee—all-natural maple syrup has about one-third fewer calories than sugar, and it's sweeter so you don't need as much.

- RAW SUGAR: Did you just fall out of your chair? Yep, sugar is okay in small doses— raw sugar, to be precise, because your body knows how to process it. This is a good option for those of you not looking to lose weight but just wanting to go a little more natural with your coffee or tea.

14

Detox Snacks for Your Sweet Tooth

A *Lose Weight by Eating* cookbook wouldn't be complete without a really extensive dessert chapter! I have a wicked sweet tooth and also believe life is too short to skip the sweet stuff. So this chapter gives lots of healthier versions of desserts and sweet treats.

While on the detox plans, you can have one of these a day as one of your snacks. By allowing yourself a treat once a day, you're less likely to blow your entire diet when you walk past a doughnut shop.

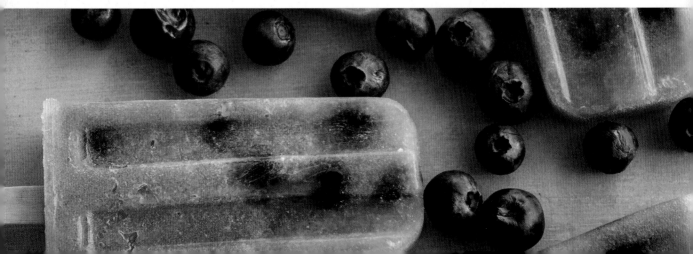

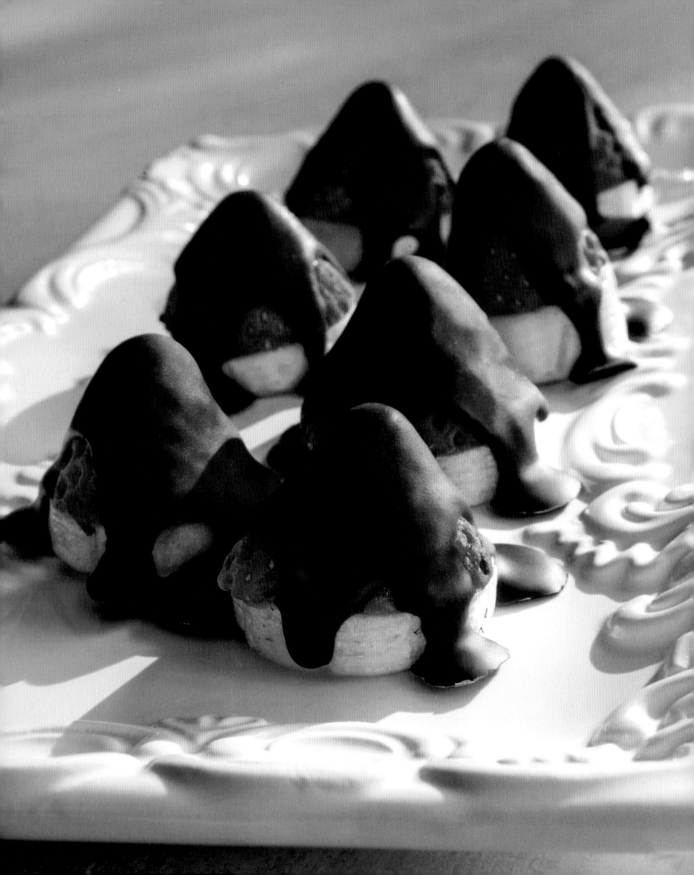

Strawberry Banana Bonbons

These are easy and delicious. Both kids and adults love them, and what's not to love about chocolate-covered fruit!

If you love chocolate as much as I do, and have the freezer space to do it, make a triple batch, and once they're frozen move them to a freezer bag. They make great sweet craving busters and are actually good for you—in moderation. Keep to the serving size; you can always have more tomorrow.

Makes 4 servings | Serving size: 2 pieces | Per serving: calories 114; fat 5 g; saturated fat 3 g; fiber 2 g; protein 1.5 g; carbohydrates 19 g; sugar 13 g | Prep time: 5 minutes plus 2 hours freeze time

1 banana
8 strawberries
¼ cup dark chocolate chips
1 teaspoon coconut oil

1. Cover a small baking sheet or large plate with parchment paper and place it in your freezer now to test out a good spot where it will stay level. You'll save yourself a lot of stress when you're dealing with melted chocolate later. Once you find a place, move the baking sheet back to your countertop.

2. Slice the banana into ½-inch-thick rounds and place them on the prepared baking sheet.

3. Slice the tops off the strawberries and place them cut side down on top of the banana rounds.

4. In a double boiler or a heatproof bowl over (but not touching) a pan filled one-third of the way with boiling water, melt the chocolate and coconut oil. Use a rubber spatula to mix gently so the chocolate doesn't burn. When the chocolate is fully melted and runny, turn off the heat and spoon it over the tops of the strawberries and bananas. You want the chocolate to drip down a little to hold the fruit together, so if need be give it a little nudge to cover the fruit.

5. Freeze for at least 2 hours before serving.

Strawberry Frozen Yogurt

Yay! I finally got an ice cream maker! So naturally I made this first, and it was so good I've made it several times since.

   If you don't have an ice cream maker and still want to try out this recipe, make it into ice pops instead (see page 50).

Makes 6 servings | Serving size: ½ cup | Per serving: calories 130;
fat 0 g; saturated fat 0 g; fiber 1 g; protein 8 g; carbohydrates 21.5 g; sugar 22 g
Prep time: 15 minutes plus 2 hours chill time and 3 hours freeze time | Cook time: 10 minutes

2 cups fresh or frozen strawberries, hulled if fresh
¼ cup raw organic sugar or coconut sugar
¼ cup pure maple syrup
2 teaspoons pure vanilla extract
2 cups 0% Greek yogurt

1. Freeze the bowl of your ice cream maker for 4 to 8 hours ahead of time (I just put it in the freezer overnight).

2. Place the strawberries, sugar, maple syrup, and vanilla in a small saucepan over medium-low heat, mixing and squishing the strawberries with the back of a wooden spoon until the sugar is melted and the strawberries are mushy and soft, about 10 minutes.

3. Remove the strawberries from the heat and add the yogurt. Mix well, then transfer to the fridge for 2 to 4 hours to cool.

4. Turn on the ice cream maker, add the chilled strawberry mixture, and let it churn for about 15 minutes, until it looks like soft serve.

5. Freeze the frozen yogurt for 2 to 3 hours, then scoop and serve. As with all ice cream/frozen yogurts, letting them sit on the counter for 10 minutes will soften them up and make scooping easier. So if you have the discipline, do so. . . .

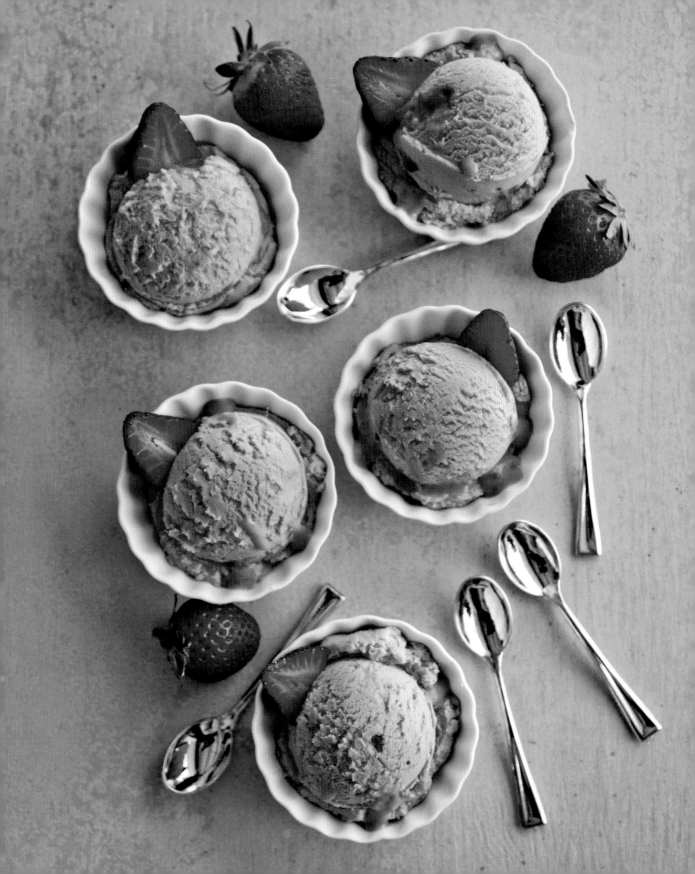

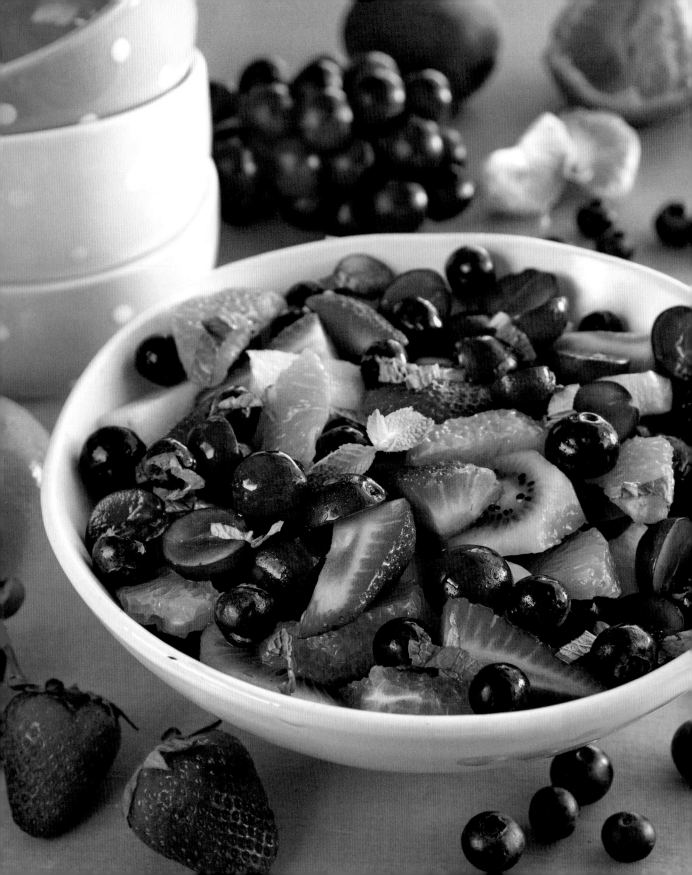

Rainbow Fruit Salad

If you're hosting or attending a brunch party, make this crowd-pleaser the night before for an easy morning. Enjoy leftovers atop yogurt, sprinkled with home-made granola (see pages 61 and 214), or portion out and freeze for a Fast Rainbow Salad Green Smoothie (recipe follows).

Makes 16 servings | Serving size: 1 cup | Per serving: calories 96; fat 0 g; saturated fat 0 g; fiber 3 g; protein 2 g; carbohydrates 24 g; sugar 18 g | Prep time: 20 minutes | Cook time: 0 minutes

1 cup fresh strawberries, hulled and quartered
1 cup clementine segments (from about
   2 clementines)
1 cup fresh pineapple, cut into bite-size cubes
1 cup cubed kiwi (from about 3 kiwis)
1 cup fresh blueberries
1 cup purple grapes, halved
½ cup roughly chopped fresh mint

DRESSING
½ cup fresh orange juice
1 tablespoon champagne vinegar
1 teaspoon honey

1. Mix together all the fruit salad ingredients in a large bowl.

2. In a small bowl, whisk together all the dressing ingredients. Drizzle the dressing over the fruit, toss well, and serve. Cover leftover fruit salad with plastic wrap and refrigerate for up to 24 hours.

Fast Rainbow Salad Green Smoothie

Turn leftovers into a smoothie with this yummy recipe!

*Per serving: calories 110; fat 0 g; saturated fat 0 g; fiber 4 g; protein 4 g; carbohydrate 26 g; sugar 18 g
Prep time: 25 minutes | Cook time: 0 minutes*

1 cup frozen leftover Rainbow Fruit Salad
2 cups spinach

Blend with ½ cup water and enjoy.

Chunky Monkey Shake

Silly name, delicious shake! This yummy banana smoothie is great for fast treats. Freeze bananas overnight so you can just dump all the ingredients into the blender and be done with it. Even if you forget to freeze the banana, it's a great shake. Just add in ½ cup ice to cool it down.

Makes 2 servings | Serving size: about 1 cup | Per serving: calories 179; fat 9 g; saturated fat 1 g; fiber 3.5 g; protein 5 g; carbohydrates 21 g; sugar 11 g | Prep time: 5 minutes | Cook time: 0 minutes

1 banana, peeled, sliced, and frozen overnight
1 cup spinach
1 tablespoon all-natural peanut butter
1 tablespoon peanuts or additional peanut butter
1 cup unsweetened almond milk

Place all the ingredients in a blender and pulse. When the mixture starts moving, blend on medium speed until smooth. Pour into a large glass and enjoy.

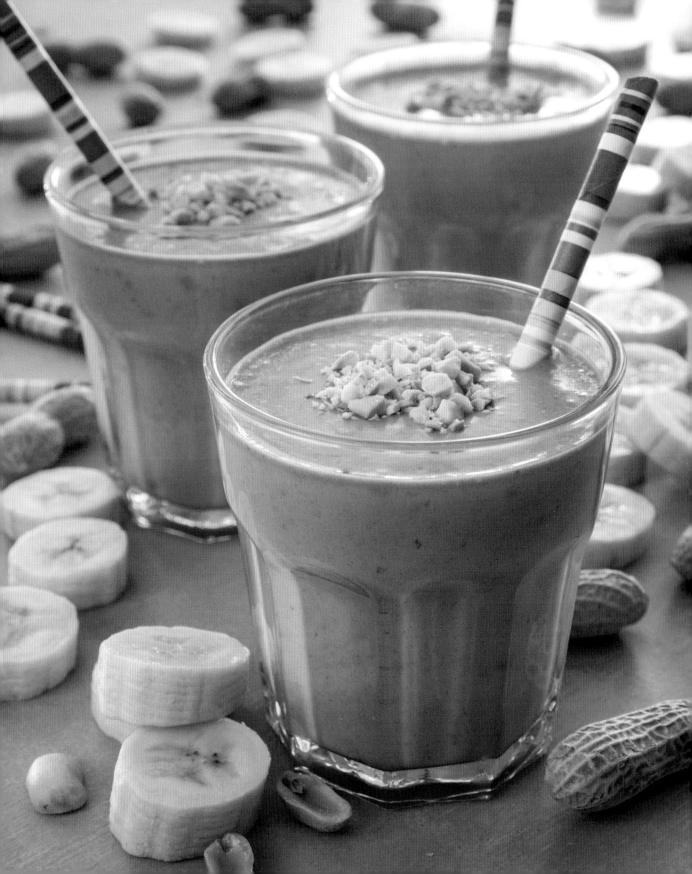

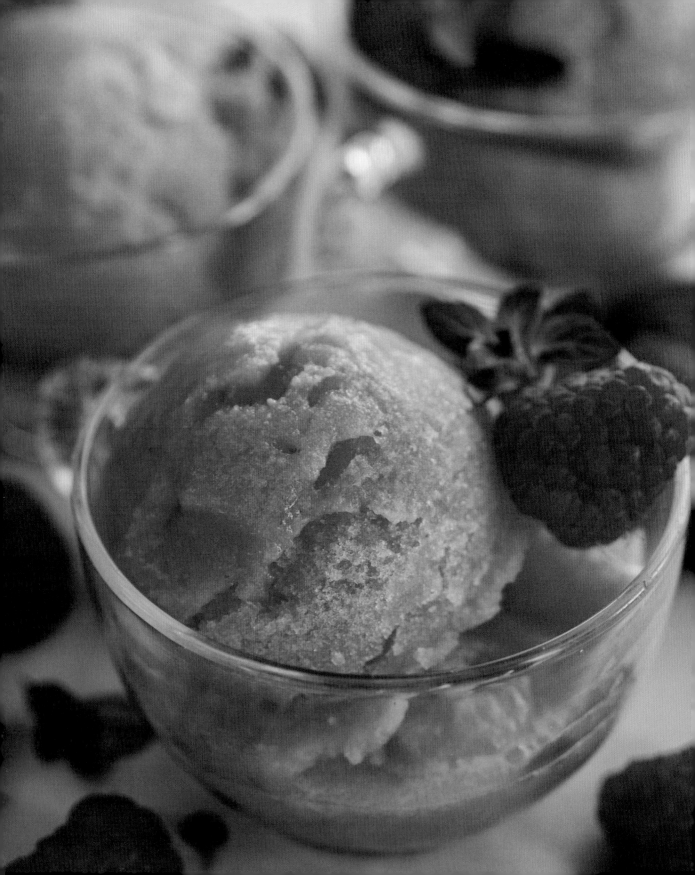

Raspberry Peach Sorbet

This sorbet is so pretty you may have a hard time digging into it. Wait, who am I kidding? You're gonna get caught eating it right from the container at 2:00 a.m., and that's okay! It's so low in calories and healthy that you can have it whenever you like.

This recipe requires no special equipment, but if you have an ice cream maker, great! Just freeze the ice cream maker bowl for 2 to 5 hours; turn it on, add the sorbet base, churn for 15 minutes, and then freeze for a couple hours.

Makes 4 servings | Serving size: about 1 cup | Per serving: calories 109; fat 0 g; saturated fat 0 g; fiber 5.5 g; protein 2 g; carbohydrates 27.5 g; sugar 20 g | Prep time: 5 minutes plus 4 hours freeze time

---

1 (10-ounce) bag frozen raspberries
1 (16-ounce) bag frozen peaches
2 tablespoons honey
1½ cups club soda

1. Clear out a spot in your freezer. You must have enough flat space on which to place a filled gallon-size bag.

2. Place all the ingredients in a blender and pulse. When the mixture starts moving, blend on medium speed until you have a smooth sorbet base.

3. Pour the sorbet into a gallon-size freezer bag and press out as much air as you can without spilling the sorbet all over the counter. Seal and place flat in the freezer for 1 hour.

4. Remove from the freezer and use a rolling pin to very carefully squish and break up the frozen chunks. Repeat this two more times: Freeze for 1 hour, squish. Freeze for 1 hour, squish.

5. Serve the sorbet or transfer it to an airtight container and pack it down well, then cover and freeze for later. It will keep in the freezer for 2 months.

Apple Snacks

This takes the boring old apple slices dipped in peanut butter to a new snack height. I swap out the peanut butter for metabolism-boosting almond butter and top it with crunchy almonds and beautifying coconut flakes. You will swoon... and your kids will try to steal them, so if you must, lock yourself in your bedroom while you snack to ward off thieving offspring.

Makes 2 servings | Serving size: ½ apple with toppings | Per serving: calories 133; fat 8 g; saturated fat 1 g; fiber 2.5 g; protein 2 g; carbohydrates 14.5 g; sugar 9 g
Prep time: 5 minutes | Cook time: 0 minutes

1 apple (I prefer Fuji, but pick your favorite)
1 tablespoon fresh lemon juice (optional)
1 tablespoon almond butter
1 teaspoon chopped unsalted almonds
1 teaspoon unsweetened coconut flakes

1. Set the apple on its side on a cutting board and slice it crosswise so you get ½-inch rings.

2. Knock the rings gently on the cutting board (so technical, I know) to dislodge the seeds. Discard the seeds. If you're packing up these snacks for later, squeeze some lemon juice over the apple slices so they don't oxidize and turn brown.

3. Smear each apple ring with a thin layer of almond butter and top with the almonds and coconut! Eat up or store in an airtight container for up to 3 days to take on the road.

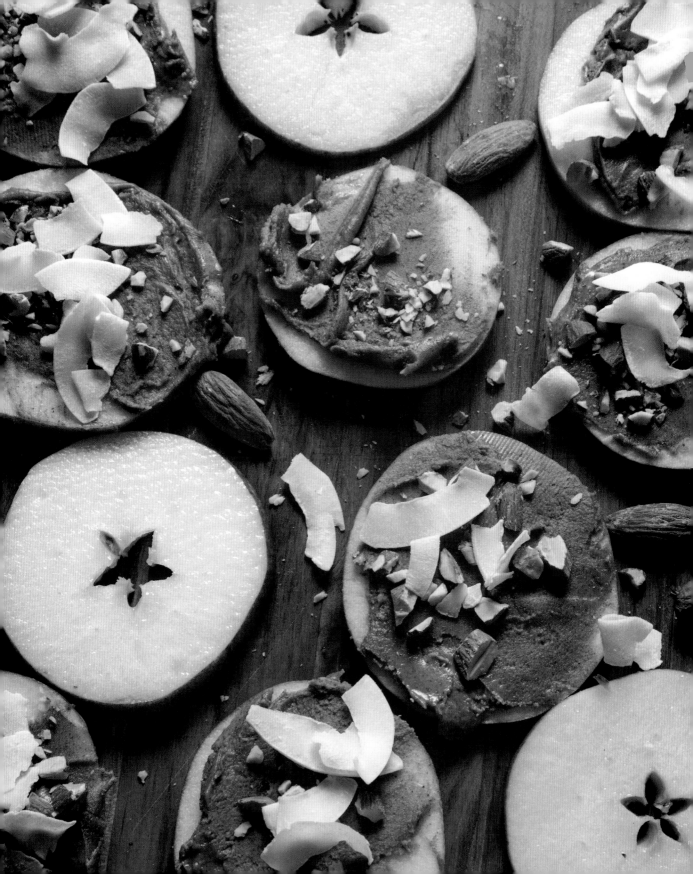

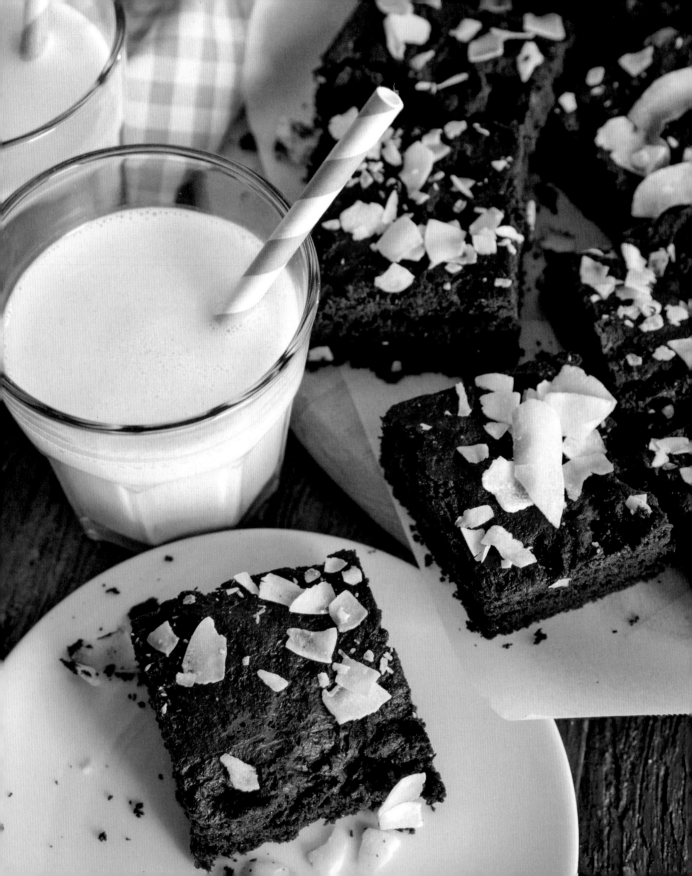

Dark Chocolate Coconut Brownies

One day after school, my daughter, Sophia, came bursting through the front door exclaiming, "Mommy, can we make brownies?" Who knows where she got the bright idea, but as a proud chocoholic, I replied with a quick *"Absolutely!"*

Because I was in the middle of testing recipes for this book, I modified the dark chocolate fudge brownies from my first cookbook and made them even healthier by taking out what little butter and sugar the recipe called for and swapping it for coconut-based ingredients. Dare I say it? . . . I think I like these even better than the original.

Makes 21 servings | Serving size: 1 brownie | Per serving: calories 148; fat 7 g; saturated fat 5 g; fiber 2 g; protein 4 g; carbohydrates 20 g; sugar 11 g | Prep time: 10 minutes | Cook time: 20 minutes

¼ cup coconut oil
1 cup dark chocolate chips
½ cup coconut sugar
1 cup 0% Greek yogurt
2 large eggs
½ cup unsweetened cocoa powder
1 teaspoon baking soda
1¼ cups all-purpose flour
½ teaspoon kosher salt
3 tablespoons unsweetened coconut flakes

1. Preheat the oven to 350°F. Line a 9 × 13-inch baking dish with parchment paper.

2. In a large saucepan, melt the coconut oil, chocolate chips, and coconut sugar over medium heat, stirring together until smooth. Remove from the heat and set aside to cool for about 5 minutes.

3. Whisk in the yogurt. At this point the mixture should be at room temperature; if not, let it sit for another 5 minutes, then whisk in the eggs until combined.

4. Whisk in the cocoa powder, baking soda, flour, and salt until you have a smooth mousse-like batter.

5. Scrape the batter into the prepared baking dish and smooth to the edges in an even layer. Sprinkle the coconut flakes over the top and bake for 20 to 25 minutes, until the outer one-third is firm to the touch and pulling away from the sides of the baking dish.

6. Let the brownies cool completely in the pan; they will continue to cook and firm up. Pull up on the parchment paper to remove the brownies from the baking dish and place them on a cutting board. Peel back the parchment paper and cut the block into 21 brownie squares (two long cuts and six short cuts).

Watermelon Ice Pops

I love how sweet watermelon can be when it's in season, so sweet that it's almost like candy. I've found that if you freeze watermelon it actually gets sweeter, which means that even if you bring home a suboptimal one, freezing it will improve the flavor. And if you're lucky enough to make this recipe when watermelon is in peak season, you'll end up with a shockingly sweet treat, with absolutely no sugar added.

Get wild blueberries if you can. They're smaller and look more like watermelon seeds. Trader Joe's has them in the frozen fruit section. But if all you have are full-size berries, these pops are equally charming and delicious.

Makes 8 servings | Serving size: 1 ice pop | Per serving: calories 22; fat 0 g; saturated fat 0 g; fiber 0.5 g; protein 0.5 g; carbohydrates 5.5 g; sugar 4.5 g | Prep time: 5 minutes plus 3 to 5 hours freeze time

---

½ cup fresh or frozen blueberries, preferably wild

3 cups cubed seeded watermelon

1. Make space in your freezer for the ice pop molds.

2. Fill each mold one-quarter of the way full of blueberries and set aside.

3. Place the watermelon in a blender and blend on high speed until smooth. Spoon the watermelon into the molds until mostly full. Use a butter knife or chopstick to gently move the berries up so they are evenly distributed throughout. Add the ice pop sticks and freeze for 3 to 5 hours.

4. To serve, let the frozen pops sit on the counter for 10 minutes, then remove them from the molds.

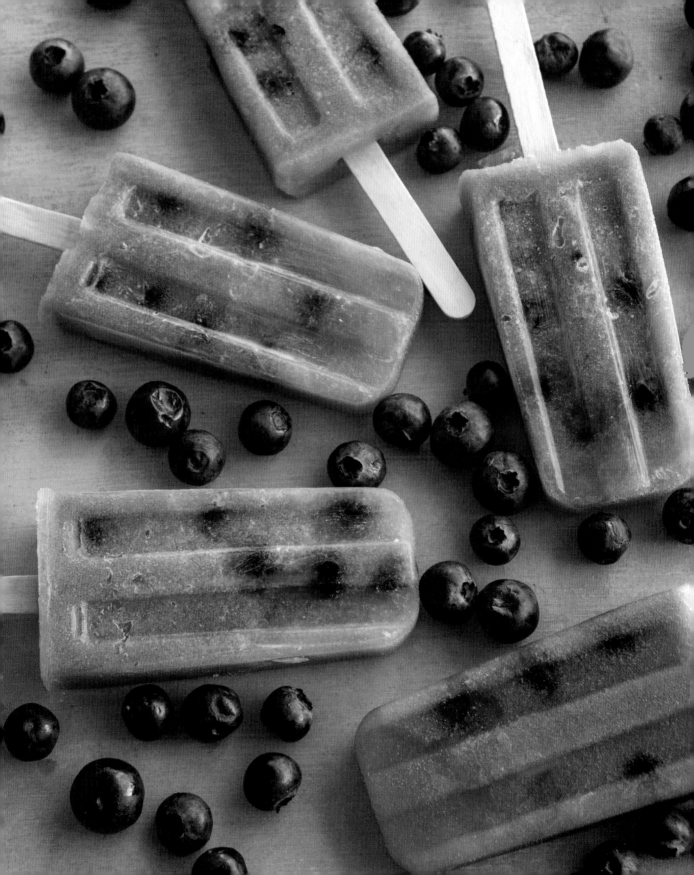

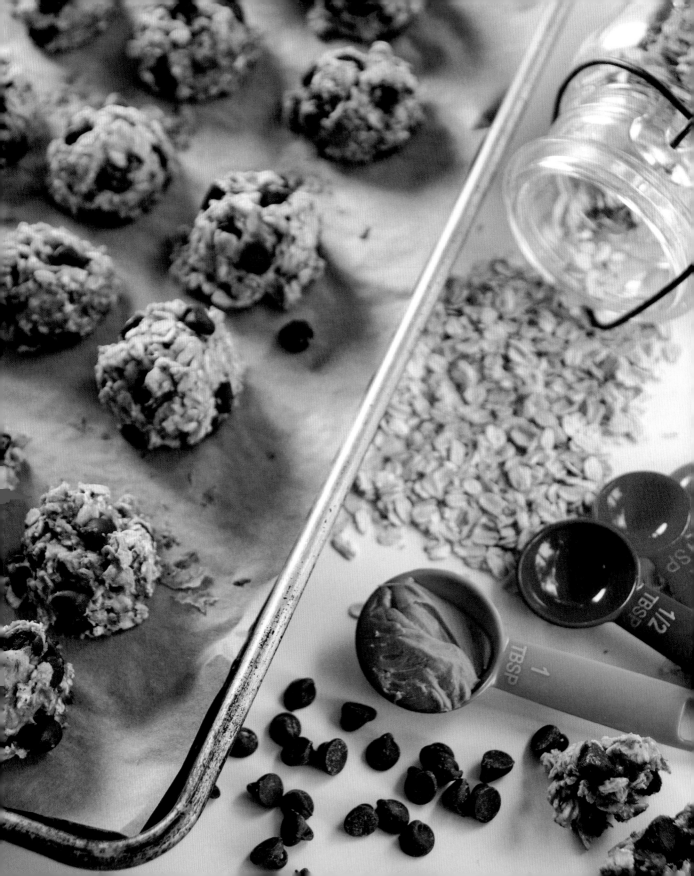

Chocolate Chip, Peanut Butter, and Banana Cookies

Wow . . . what a mouthful! But this recipe name is fitting as you're going to have a mouthful of chocolate chip goodness until these are all gone. So do yourself a favor and plan on giving some away, or freeze half the batch—they're seriously addictive!

These yummy vegan cookies are free of butter, added sugar, and even eggs—the peanut butter and applesauce hold them together. But trust me when I say you won't miss the sugar. The sweet banana and abundance of chocolate more than make up for it.

Makes 24 cookies | Serving size: 1 cookie | Per serving: calories 79; fat 3 g; saturated fat 1 g; fiber 1.5 g; protein 2 g; carbohydrates 13.5 g; sugar 4.5 g | Prep time: 15 minutes | Cook time: 10 minutes

---

¾ cup all-purpose flour
½ teaspoon kosher salt
½ teaspoon baking soda
1 banana, thinly sliced
2 tablespoons all-natural peanut butter
½ cup unsweetened applesauce
1 teaspoon pure vanilla extract
2 cups old-fashioned rolled oats
⅔ cup semisweet chocolate chips

1. Preheat the oven to 350°F. Line two baking sheets with parchment paper.

2. In a medium bowl, whisk together the flour, salt, and baking soda.

3. In a large bowl, mash together the banana, peanut butter, applesauce, and vanilla with the back of a fork. Whisk in ⅓ cup water, scrape the sides, and mix well.

4. Add the flour mixture to the banana mixture and stir together until just combined. Stir in the oats and chocolate chips.

5. Use a small ice cream scoop or spoon to drop Ping-Pong ball–size dollops of cookie dough onto the prepared baking sheets. They don't spread much, so you only need ½ inch of space between the cookies. Bake for 10 minutes, or until lightly browned on the bottom. Let them cool on the baking sheet for 10 minutes before devouring. You can freeze baked cookies in a gallon-size freezer bag for up to 3 months.

Mini Pumpkin Scones with Chocolate Pecan Glaze

This recipe comes toward the end of the Sweet Tooth chapter, as they're a treat, not something for every day . . . just a little gift to you. They're a chocolaty delight that's far lower in calories, sugar, and fat than the average treat, but with the amount of sugar in the recipe these should be a once-a-week treat, unlike the other once-a-day treats in this chapter.

I have cut as much sugar out of these as possible, but they do still contain sugar, so eat in moderation! The good news is that they freeze wonderfully, which really helps for portion control.

Makes 24 servings | Serving size: 1 mini scone | Per serving: calories 129; fat 5 g; saturated fat 2 g; fiber 1 g; protein 2 g; carbohydrates 20 g; sugar 7 g | Prep time: 10 minutes | Cook time: 15 minutes

SCONES
3 cups all-purpose flour
½ cup raw organic sugar
1 teaspoon baking soda
1 teaspoon baking powder
1 teaspoon pumpkin pie spice
½ teaspoon kosher salt
4 tablespoons (½ stick) cold unsalted butter
½ cup pumpkin puree
½ cup unsweetened almond milk

GLAZE
½ cup dark chocolate chips
1 teaspoon coconut oil
3 tablespoons finely chopped pecans

1. Make the scones: Preheat the oven to 375°F. Line a baking sheet with parchment paper.

2. In a large bowl or standing mixer, whisk together the flour, sugar, baking soda, baking powder, pumpkin pie spice, and salt. Cut the butter into small pieces and add it to the flour mixture, working it together with your fingers until the chunks are as small as peas.

3. In a small bowl, whisk together the pumpkin puree and almond milk. Slowly add to the flour mixture, mixing until just combined.

4. Flour a clean surface and turn out the dough. Split into 3 dough balls on the floured surface.

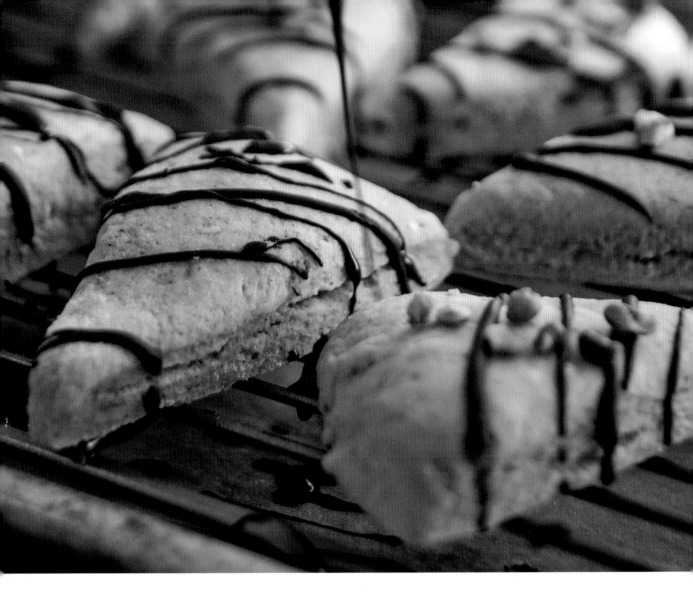

5. Gently press the dough into 3 discs, each about 1 inch thick. Using a pizza cutter, cut each disc into 8 wedges, just as if you were cutting a pizza or a pie.

6. Arrange the wedges on the prepared baking sheet; they can be close together but shouldn't touch. Bake for 10 to 15 minutes, until slightly golden.

7. Let the scones cool on the baking sheet for 5 minutes (they will continue cooking a little).

8. Make the glaze: In a double boiler or a heatproof bowl over (but not touching) a pan filled one-third of the way with boiling water, melt the chocolate chips and coconut oil. Use a rubber spatula to mix gently so the chocolate doesn't burn. Drizzle the chocolate glaze over the cooled scones and immediately sprinkle the pecans on top so they stick to the chocolate. Let cool for 10 minutes to allow the chocolate to set. Store leftover scones in a gallon-size freezer bag and freeze for up to 3 months.

Frozen Hot Chocolate

A few years back my mother-in-law sent me some frozen hot chocolate mix from Serendipity in New York. It was delicious but also so expensive that she told me, "Enjoy—that's all you get!" So I had to come up with my own homemade recipe, and I just so happened to cut hundreds of calories when I did.

So I guess you could say this was a very serendipitous recipe!

Makes 2 servings | Serving size: 8 ounces | Per serving: calories 133; fat 7 g; saturated fat 4 g; fiber 2 g; protein 2 g; carbohydrates 20 g; sugar 16.5 g | Prep time: 10 minutes | Cook time: 5 minutes

3 tablespoons semisweet chocolate chips
1 teaspoon unsweetened cocoa powder
1 teaspoon honey
½ cup unsweetened almond milk

1. In a small saucepan over medium-low heat, stir together the chocolate chips, cocoa powder, honey, and almond milk. Stir constantly until the chocolate chips melt. Remove from the heat and refrigerate for 10 minutes to cool to room temperature.

2. Scrape the chocolate sauce into a blender, top with 1 cup ice, and blend until smooth. Serve immediately (but try not to drink directly out of the blender).

15

Detox Snacks

Finally, the snack chapter! While on these detox plans, you can have as many veggies as you like. Really, go crazy with the veggies! Not a fan of veggies? Well, here I give you four dips to help you enjoy them better. So pick your favorite veggies and dig into some yummy Homemade Hummus or Hot Spinach Cheese Dip.

Choose one or two of these snacks each day to keep your metabolism roaring between meals and your tummy full and happy.

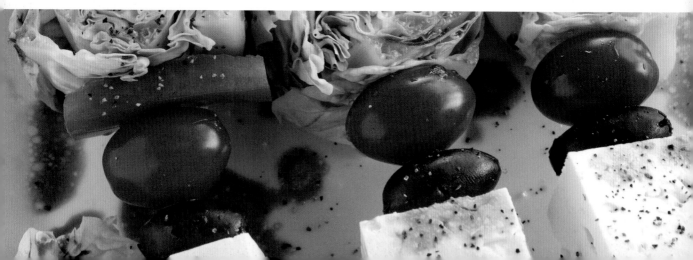

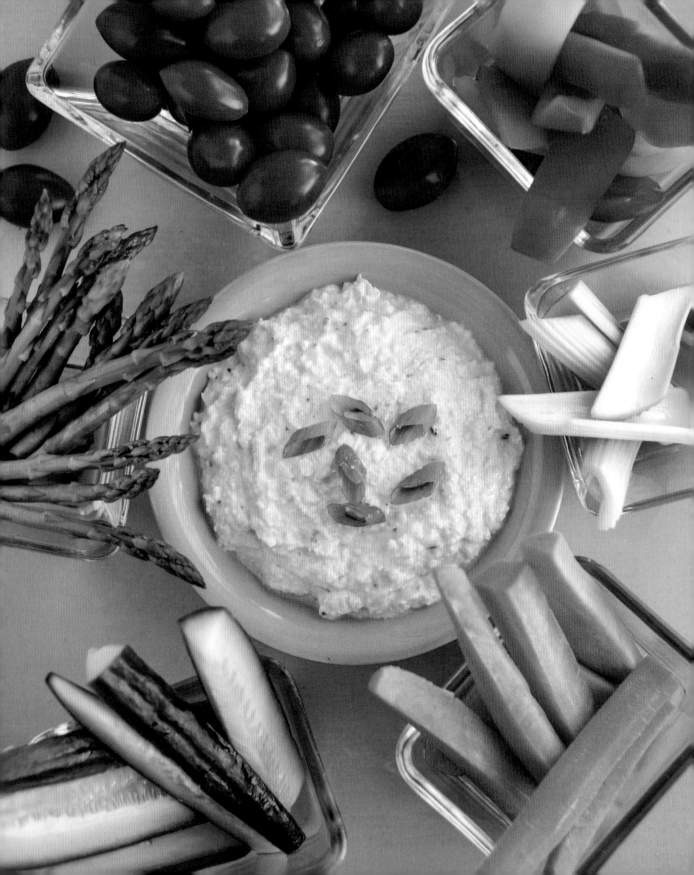

French Onion Dip with Veggie Sticks

I always have a huge tub of Greek yogurt in my fridge, sometimes two. . . . So dips happen a lot in my house. They're a great way to get your family to eat raw veggies, and with ingredients like Greek yogurt, you're also giving them a healthy boost of calcium and protein.

Makes 4 servings | Serving size: ¼ cup dip and 1 cup veggies | Per serving: calories 117; fat 4 g; saturated fat 1.5 g; fiber 2 g; protein 9.5 g; carbohydrates 13 g; sugar 7.5 g
Prep time: 10 minutes | Cook time: 60 minutes

2 medium yellow onions
Olive oil spray
Kosher salt
Leaves from 2 fresh thyme sprigs
1 garlic clove, minced
5 drops Worcestershire sauce
1 cup 0% Greek yogurt
2 tablespoons finely grated Gruyère cheese
Pinch of freshly ground black pepper
4 cups mixed veggie sticks (I like cucumber and
  red bell pepper with this)

1. Use a mandoline to slice the onions as thinly as you can. Lightly spray a large skillet with oil spray, add the onions and a pinch of salt, and stir to mix. Turn the heat to medium-low and cook very slowly for 45 minutes, stirring often to avoid burning. If they start burning, turn down the heat to low.

2. Add the thyme and garlic and cook for 15 minutes more. When the onions are browned, sticky, and beautifully caramelized, stir in the Worcestershire and turn off the heat.

3. Combine the onions, yogurt, and cheese in a food processor and blend until smooth. Taste and add the pepper and another small pinch of salt, as needed. Serve with the veggie sticks.

Chips and Salsa and Guacamole, Oh My!

Sometimes you just need some chips and salsa. I get it, trust me! So here's a healthy version with some whole wheat chips *and* veggies to dip and enjoy your goodies.

So why the veggies? Because if you ate only chips here, that would be too many carbs for a daily healthy snack. But swap half the chips for some veggies and voilà, you have a healthy snack. And let's be honest here—it's usually the crunch you're looking for when you crave chips, so these crunchy veggies will hit the spot.

Makes 2 servings | Serving size: 6 chips, ½ cup salsa, ¼ cup guacamole, and as many carrots and bell peppers as you like! | Per serving: calories 143; fat 7 g; saturated fat 1 g; fiber 5 g; protein 4.5 g; carbohydrates 17 g; sugar 20 g | Prep time: 20 minutes | Cook time: 10 minutes

CHIPS
1 (8-inch) whole wheat tortilla
1 teaspoon olive oil
¼ teaspoon kosher salt
¼ teaspoon garlic powder

SALSA
2 large tomatoes, chopped
¼ red onion, minced
1 jalapeño, ribs and seeds removed, minced
2 tablespoons chopped fresh cilantro
Juice of ½ lime
Kosher salt and freshly ground black pepper

GUACAMOLE
1 avocado
¼ cup 0% Greek yogurt
Juice of ½ lime
3 tablespoons salsa (recipe above)

VEGGIE STICKS
1 red bell pepper, sliced into thick strips
1 carrot, cut into thin rings on the diagonal

1. Make the chips: Preheat the oven to 425°F.

2. Brush both sides of the tortilla with the oil and sprinkle with the salt and garlic powder. Use a pizza wheel, sharp knife, or scissors to cut the tortilla into 12 wedges, just as you would cut a pizza or pie.

3. Transfer the wedges to a baking sheet and bake for about 10 minutes, until slightly crispy. They'll crisp up more as they cool.

4. Make the salsa: Mix together all the ingredients in a small bowl. (Do it a day ahead for maximum flavor.)

5. Make the guacamole: In a small bowl, smash the avocado with the back of a fork until you reach the desired consistency. Mix in the yogurt, lime, and salsa. If taking in your lunch box, move to an airtight container and squeeze more lime over the top; this will stop it from browning quickly.

6. Place the veggies and chips on a plate and the salsa and guacamole in small bowls or ramekins (or place everything in separate airtight containers for your lunch box). Dig in and enjoy . . . and have more veggies if you like!

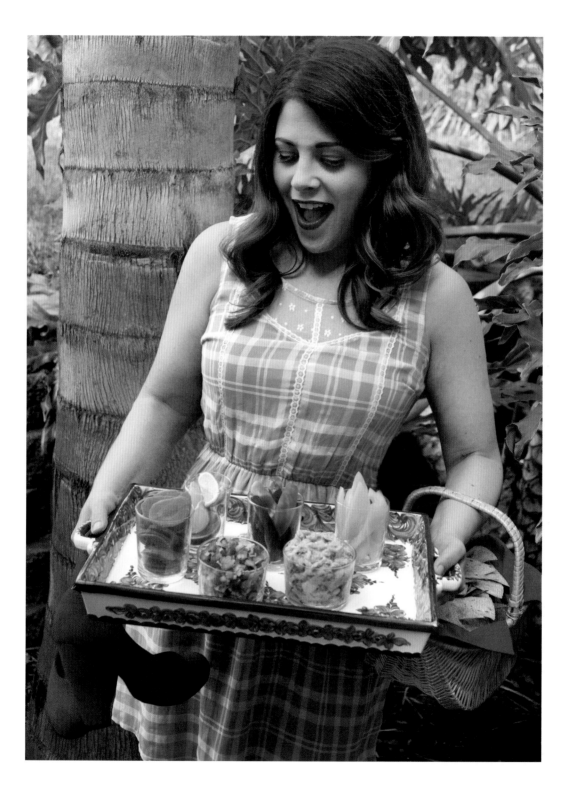

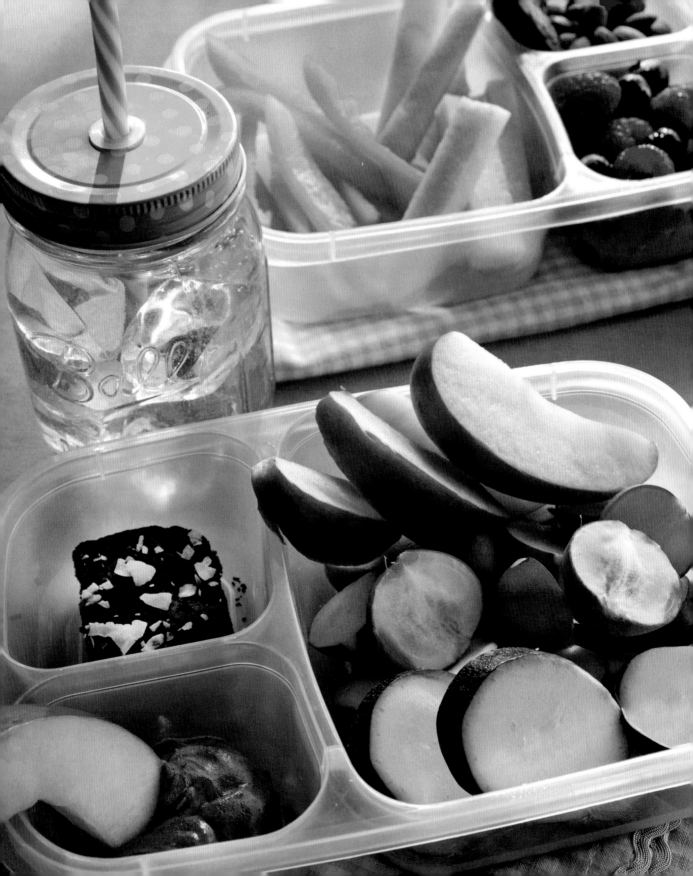

Snack Boxes

I'd hardly call this a recipe, more like tips on how to set up the perfect snack for your lunch box, or for enjoying on the couch. You choose—in fact, you get to choose everything!

I recommend getting a compartmentalized (wow, I spelled that right on the first try!) travel container so that you can fill it up each day with your goodies and so that they stay fresh and in their individual spots. If you don't have one, simply layer the snacks with parchment paper in whatever travel container is available.

Prep time: 1 to 5 minutes | Cook time: 0 to 15 minutes

VEGGIES (PICK 2)
1 red bell pepper, sliced into strips
2 celery stalks, trimmed and halved
½ cucumber, sliced into rings
1 endive, trimmed into individual leaves
1 jicama, peeled and sliced into sticks (1 serving is 3 sticks)
5 radishes, trimmed and halved
1 zucchini, sliced into ¼-inch-thick rings

FRUIT (PICK 1)
5 strawberries, hulled and halved
1 banana
1 apple, cored, sliced, and sprinkled with lemon juice (to keep it from turning brown)
1 pear, cored and quartered
1 orange, peeled and segmented
⅓ cup berries, such as blueberries, blackberries, raspberries, or a combo
⅓ cup grapes
1 kiwi, quartered
⅓ cup mango slices
⅓ cup cubed pineapple
⅓ cup cubed melon (watermelon, honeydew, cantaloupe)

PROTEIN (PICK 1)
2 tablespoons unsalted nuts
2 tablespoons raw nut butter (to dip those apples and celery in!)
1 piece organic string cheese
2 tablespoons cubed cheese
½ cooked chicken breast, sliced

TREAT (PICK 1)
1 tablespoon dark chocolate chips
2 dates
1 teaspoon honey (to pour over your fruit)
1 dessert (from chapter 14)

The rest is simple—just set up your snack box, and enjoy! Try to switch it up weekly so that you don't get bored with the same old, same old.

Greek Salad Skewers

Oh, yum, I really *love* these! And this delivery method makes a salad so much more fun. (Yep, I'm trying to trick you into eating salad!)

Now, I know these are in the snack section, and they *do* make excellent snacks, but if you're getting all the ingredients for these, you might as well trick your family into eating salad, too, right? These are great as a side with dinner; pair them with some baked chicken and asparagus and you have a perfect detox meal. This snack is so versatile. You're welcome! (*wink*)

Makes 3 servings | Serving size: 1 skewer | Per serving: calories 102; fat 6 g; saturated fat 2 g; fiber 5 g; protein 5 g; carbohydrates 10 g; sugar 4 g | Prep time: 15 minutes | Cook time: 0 minutes

DRESSING

½ teaspoon extra-virgin olive oil
1 tablespoon balsamic vinegar
2 tablespoons fresh lemon juice
Kosher salt and freshly ground black pepper

SALAD SKEWERS

1 romaine heart
½ red bell pepper, cut into 6 bite-size chunks
3 cherry tomatoes
3 pitted Kalamata olives
3 peperoncini (optional)
3 tablespoon-size cubes feta cheese

1. Place all the dressing ingredients in a mason jar with a tight-fitting lid or small bowl, and shake or whisk vigorously to combine.

2. Slide a chunk of bell pepper onto each skewer to start. Cut off the bottom of the romaine heart and skewer it, leaving about ½ inch of lettuce on one side of the skewer. Slide the lettuce to the bottom of the skewer, then cut off the rest of the romaine head so that you're left with a 1-inch-thick disc

of lettuce on the skewer. A lettuce lollipop! Do this on all three skewers (this helps keep the romaine together; some will fall onto the cutting board but that's okay—you'll still use it). Continue sliding the bell pepper and romaine onto the skewer until you have three layers.

3. Add a cherry tomato, then an olive, then a peperoncino (if using). Carefully slide on the cheese so the cube stays together (feta can be crumbly).

4. Give the dressing another shake, then drizzle over the skewers, paying special attention to the romaine—make sure it really gets in between the leaves for best flavor.

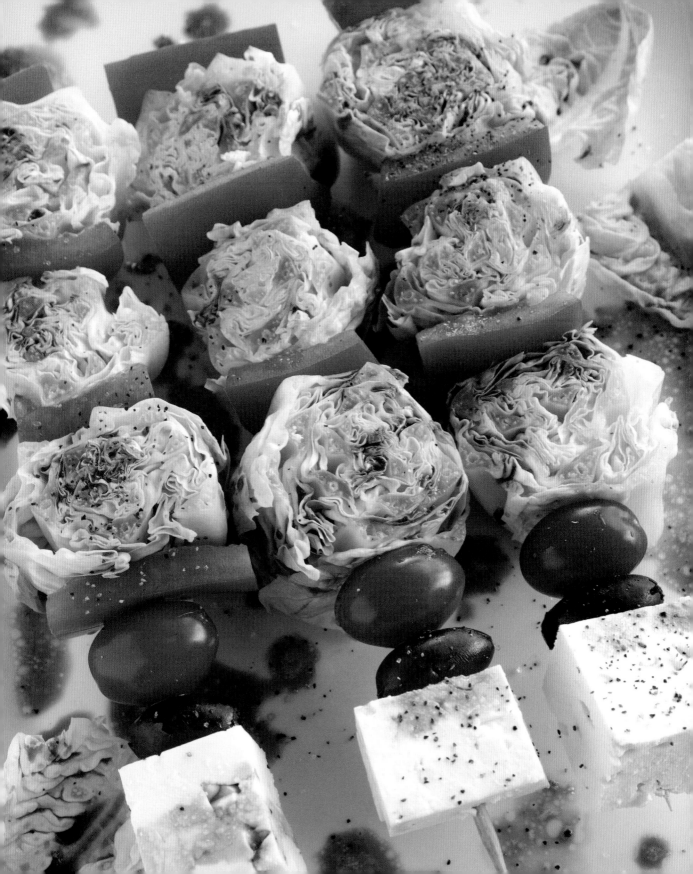

Hot Spinach Cheese Dip with Veggie Sticks

I used to film how-to cooking videos for eHow, and this is one of my favorite recipes from my videos!

This dip is great for get-togethers, potlucks, and even game day. I like to serve it with veggie sticks—they offer such a satisfying crunch that I never miss the chips—and you can have as many veggie sticks as you like, which is something you can't say about chips!

Makes 6 servings | *Serving size: ¼ cup dip and as many veggies as you like* | *Per serving: calories 168; fat 11 g; saturated fat 6 g; fiber 1 g; protein 8.5 g; carbohydrates 10 g; sugar 5 g*
Prep time: 10 minutes | *Cook time: 25 minutes*

2 tablespoons unsalted butter
2 tablespoons all-purpose flour
2½ cups unsweetened almond milk
2 garlic cloves
4 cups chopped fresh spinach
¾ cup grated low-fat sharp cheddar cheese
¼ cup freshly grated Parmesan cheese
½ cup 0% Greek yogurt
3 to 5 cups veggie sticks, such as bell pepper, carrot, celery, cucumber, and/or zucchini

1. Melt the butter in a large saucepan over medium heat, add the flour, and whisk together with a wooden spoon for about 5 minutes, until you have a lightly browned paste (this is a roux).

2. Pour in the almond milk and whisk until combined. Add the garlic cloves and stir often until the sauce thickens and coats the back of the spoon, about 15 minutes. Remove the garlic and discard.

3. Stir in the spinach; it will wilt and darken. When the spinach is wilted and reduced by half, about 5 minutes, remove the pan from the heat and stir in the cheeses. Add the yogurt, stir again, then transfer to a serving bowl. Serve hot with the veggie sticks and enjoy! Store leftover dip in the refrigerator for up to 3 days. Reheat in a saucepan before serving.

Pita Pizza Triangles

These are a big hit in my house. I make them whenever the neighborhood kids come over, which is often! Sure, the recipe is meant to be for you and me, but there is certainly no harm in the kiddos liking them as well!

   If you do decide to make them for your little ones, let them top their own triangles. Less work for you, fewer complaints from them.

*Makes 4 servings | Serving size: **4 triangles** | Per serving: calories 118; fat 4 g; saturated fat 2 g; fiber 3 g; protein 6 g; carbohydrates 16 g; sugar 5 g | Prep time: 10 minutes | Cook time: 10 minutes*

2 whole wheat pitas
1 cup homemade marinara sauce (see page 155) or organic store-bought
½ cup shredded mozzarella cheese
1 green onion, thinly sliced
2 tablespoons minced fresh pineapple
¼ cup minced white mushrooms
¼ cup minced red bell pepper

1. Preheat the oven to 350°F.

2. Cut the pitas into quarters, open the pockets, and cut along the seam so that you have 8 triangles per pita half (16 total). Place them on two rimmed baking sheets.

3. Toast the pita triangles in the oven for 5 minutes. Remove from the oven, but leave the oven on.

4. Top each triangle with 2 tablespoons of the sauce and 1½ teaspoons of the cheese; then you can have fun topping them. I like to top one-third of the triangles with green onion and pineapple, one-third with mushroom and bell pepper, and one-third with everything.

5. Place them on the baking sheets and bake for about 5 minutes, until the cheese is melted.

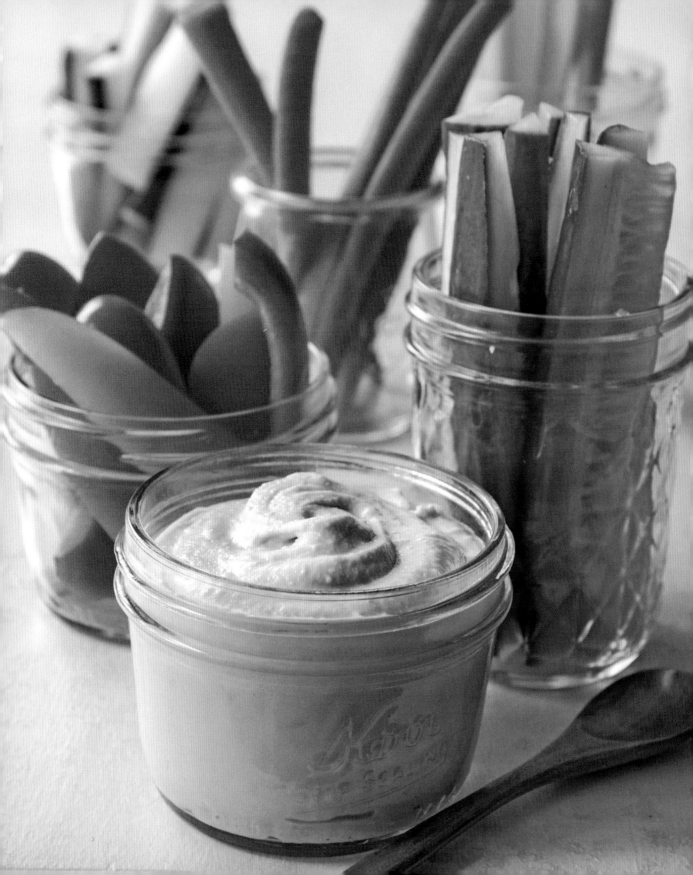

Homemade Hummus with Veggie Sticks

I can't tell you how many times I've made hummus at home, just to be disappointed in the results. I've tried dozens of recipes and they always come out grainy or too runny, or they use so much oil that you feel as if you're snacking on salad dressing.

Well, I came across a tip that changed all of that—use the liquid from the can of chickpeas! This changed everything for me, giving me a creamy, perfect hummus. Try this trick and never overspend on store-bought hummus again.

Makes 3 servings | Serving size: ⅓ cup hummus and as many veggies as you want!
Per serving: calories 196; fat 8 g; saturated fat 1 g; fiber 9 g; protein 10 g;
carbohydrates 34 g; sugar 6 g | Prep time: 15 minutes | Cook time: 0 minutes

---

1 (15-ounce) can chickpeas (garbanzo beans)
2 garlic cloves
3 tablespoons fresh lemon juice
2 tablespoons tahini
Kosher salt and freshly ground black pepper
3 to 5 cups veggie sticks, such as bell pepper, carrot, celery, cucumber, and zucchini

1. Drain the liquid from the chickpeas into a small bowl.

2. Place the chickpeas, half of the bean liquid, the garlic, lemon juice, tahini, and a pinch each of salt and black pepper in a blender. Blend until smooth, adding more of the bean liquid as needed to thin it out.

3. Taste for seasoning and add more salt and pepper as needed, then transfer to a serving bowl. Serve with as many veggie sticks as you like!

Acknowledgments

Writing a book takes a village, and my village is filled with amazing people! Thank you to my family, Chris and Sophia, for believing in me and encouraging me to follow my dreams. You helped me test recipes, took work off my plate to give me time to write, and even went grocery shopping when I was elbow deep in a recipe test and missing a single ingredient.

To my extended family, for always being so supportive, cheering me on, and inspiring me.

To my best friend of thirty years, Kara Dowling: I leaned on you the most during this long process. Thank you for always being there for me and for being the best sister, friend, and soul mate a gal could ever ask for!

To my amazing editor, Cassie Jones: I'm honored to be one of your authors and to work with you! To the entire HarperCollins team, for helping me make this book the best it can be. To my agents, Sarah Passick and Celeste Fine, for believing in me and helping me make this book happen.

To my photography team—my amazing amazing team—I adore you! You helped me turn black-and-white pages into a colorful masterpiece. Cindy Epstein, your food styling is art! I feel so blessed to know you and call you my friend. Carl Kravats, your photographs are brilliant and your use of light in all these wonderful pictures astounds me! Joni Wilhelm, our kitchen goddess, thank you so much for all your hard work, for testing all the recipes, and for helping make this book so beautiful.

Many friends and family members helped me test recipes for the book as well. To my sister-in-law, Brenda Johns, thank you for contributing an amazing recipe to the book—your ceviche is legendary. Kate Klein, thank you for helping me create a wonderful smoothie inspired by your award-winning pie and for inspiring me years ago to get in the kitchen. To my childhood friend Chef Ted Hill, thank you for helping me test the shrimp recipes for the book. Rachel Plummer, thank you for helping me re-create our old favorite lunch date meal. Marilinda Schor, thank you for helping me test the last few recipes. Thank you to all the friends, family, and readers who helped me test the quiz and programs. And a big thank you to Katie Read, for bravely testing the pregnancy/nursing program days after your new bundle of joy came into the world—like you didn't already have enough going on!

Thank you to all my readers. It's such a thrill to put a book out into the world and know people are enjoying it. Many of you made requests after the last book, and I did my best to incorporate all of them in this book. And I'll do it again and again and again, for as long as the publishing world will have me.

Last, a note to all the brave women and little girls out there. We are strong, so much stronger than we give ourselves credit for. Be fearless, break the mold, shatter the glass ceiling, and never let anyone tell you your dreams are unrealistic. Be kind to one another and support your sisters—kindness is beauty!

Healthy Food Benefits

I took the most-used ingredients in this book and outlined their health benefits, so if you have a migraine or feel bloated, you can look up the ingredients that will help you feel better faster.

FRUITS

Açaí   Vitamin A. Boosts the immune system; supports healthy skin and eyes

Apples   Fiber and vitamin C. Promote healthy heart and younger-looking skin; increases metabolism and energy

Bananas   Fiber, vitamins C and B_6, potassium, and manganese. Promote a healthy heart, skin, bones, immune and nervous systems; increase metabolism and energy; reduce stress

Blueberries   Fiber and vitamins C and K: Promote healthy heart and younger-looking skin; increase metabolism; regulate blood sugar; reduce bone loss

Cherries   Fiber and vitamins A and C. Promote healthy heart, skin, eyes; boost immune system; reduce pain

Citrus (oranges, limes, lemons)   Potassium, fiber, and vitamin C. Promotes healthy bones, heart, muscles, nervous system; increases metabolism; promotes younger-looking skin

Cranberries   Vitamins E, K, and C and fiber. Contain anti-aging properties; balance hormones; increase metabolism; thicken hair; regulate blood sugar

Grapes   Vitamins C and K. Increase energy; promote younger-looking skin

Kiwis   Fiber; vitamins E, C, and K; and potassium. Contain anti-aging properties; balance hormones; increase metabolism; thicken hair; promote strong bones and muscles

Mangoes   Fiber; vitamins E, C, and K; and potassium. Promote healthy heart, bones, muscles, and younger-looking skin; increase metabolism; regulate blood sugar; reduce bone loss

Peaches   Fiber, vitamins A and C, niacin, and potassium. Promote a healthy heart, skin, eyes, bones, muscles; increase energy and metabolism; promote younger-looking skin

Pineapples   Fiber, thiamin, and vitamins B_6 and C. Promote healthy heart, skin, immune system and memory; increase metabolism

Pomegranates   Folate, potassium, and vitamin K. Promote healthy heart, muscles, nervous system, and bones; reduce stress

Raspberries   Vitamin K, magnesium, fiber, vitamin C, and manganese. Promote strong bones and a healthy heart; reduce pain, migraines, and inflammation; increase metabolism and energy

Strawberries   Folate, potassium, fiber, vitamin C, and manganese. Promote healthy heart, muscles, bones, and nervous system; reduce stress; increase metabolism and energy

Tomatoes   Vitamins E, A, C, K, and B_6; thiamin; niacin; folate; magnesium; fiber; potassium; and manganese. Contain anti-aging properties; balance hormones; reduce stress; promote healthy skin, eyes, hair, heart, and bones

Watermelons   Potassium and vitamins A and C. Promote strong bones, muscles, and immune system; promote healthy skin, eyes, and younger-looking skin

VEGETABLES

Arugula   Vitamins A and K, folate, and potassium. Boosts immune system; promotes healthy skin, eyes, heart, bones, and muscles; reduces bone loss; regulates blood sugar

Asparagus   Calcium; magnesium; zinc; fiber; vitamins A, C, E, K, and B_6; thiamin; riboflavin; niacin; folate; iron; and potassium. Promotes healthy bones, muscles, heart, immune system, skin, eyes, hair, and nervous system; contains anti-aging properties; improves memory

Bell peppers   Thiamin; niacin; folate; magnesium; fiber; vitamins A, C, K, and B_6; potassium; and manganese. Contain anti-aging properties; improve memory; lower

cholesterol; promote healthy heart, bones, and muscles; increase metabolism; reduce stress

Broccoli   thiamin; niacin; calcium; iron; vitamins A, C, and B_6; riboflavin, folate; magnesium; potassium; and manganese. Contains anti-aging properties; improves memory; promotes healthy heart, bones, muscles, skin, eyes, immune system, and nervous system; reduces inflammation

Brussels sprouts   Riboflavin; iron; magnesium; phosphorus; fiber, vitamins A, C, K, and B_6; thiamin; folate, potassium; and manganese. Strengthen immune system, bones, muscles, and heart; prevent acne; increase metabolism and energy

Butternut squash   Fiber; vitamin E; thiamin; niacin; vitamin B_6, A, and C; folate; calcium; magnesium; potassium; and manganese. Promotes healthy heart, skin, immune system, muscles, bones, eyes, and nervous system

Cabbage   Thiamin; calcium; iron; magnesium; potassium; fiber; vitamins C, K, and B_6; folate; and manganese. Contains anti-aging properties; improves memory; prevents PMS; promotes healthy bones, muscles, and immune system

Carrots   Thiamin; niacin; vitamins B_6, A, C, and K; folate; manganese; fiber; potassium. Contain anti-aging properties; improve memory; lower cholesterol; promote healthy heart, skin, immune system, bones, eyes, and nervous system

Celery   Riboflavin; vitamins B_6, A, C, and K; calcium; magnesium; fiber; folate; potassium; and manganese. Strengthens immune and nervous system; prevents acne; reduces stress; increases metabolism; promotes healthy heart and bones

Cucumbers   Vitamins A, C, and K; magnesium; phosphorus; manganese; and potassium. Boost immune system; promote healthy skin, eyes, and bones; reduce inflammation

Eggplants   Vitamins C, K, and B$_6$; thiamin; niacin; magnesium; fiber; folate; potassium; and manganese. Increase energy and metabolism; promote younger-looking skin, healthy heart, bones, and muscles; improve memory

Jalapeños   Riboflavin; niacin; iron; magnesium; fiber; vitamins A, C, K, and B$_6$; thiamin; folate; potassium; and manganese. Contain anti-aging properties; strengthen immune system; promote healthy heart and muscles; reduce inflammation and stress

Kale   Fiber; thiamin; riboflavin; folate; iron; magnesium; vitamins A, C, K, and B$_6$; calcium; potassium; and manganese. Promotes healthy heart, muscles, bones, eyes, skin, and immune system; contains anti-aging properties; improves memory; increases metabolism

Mushrooms   Fiber, vitamin C, folate, iron, zinc, manganese, vitamins D and B$_6$, thiamin, riboflavin, niacin, phosphorus, and potassium. Promote healthy heart, muscles, eyes, bones, immune and nervous systems, and skin; decrease pain, inflammation, and stress

Onions   Fiber, vitamins B$_6$ and C, folate, potassium, and manganese. Promote healthy heart, skin, immune system, muscles, and bones; increase metabolism; reduce stress and inflammation

Parsnips   Potassium, fiber, vitamins C and K, folate, and manganese. Promote strong bones, muscles, nervous system, and heart; reduce stress and bone loss; promote younger-looking skin

Potatoes   Fiber, vitamins B$_6$ and C, and potassium. Promote healthy heart, bones, muscles, skin, and immune system; increase metabolism and energy

Romaine lettuce   Riboflavin; vitamin B$_6$, A, C, and K; calcium; magnesium; fiber; thiamin; folate; iron; potassium; and manganese. Contains anti-aging properties; strengthens immune system; prevents acne; reduces stress and fatigue; increases metabolism

Spinach   Niacin; zinc; fiber; vitamins A, C, E, K, and B$_6$; thiamin; riboflavin; folate; calcium; iron; magnesium; potassium; and manganese. Lowers cholesterol; clears up acne; improves memory; boosts immune system; promotes healthy immune system, heart, muscles, and bones

Zucchini   Vitamins A, C, K, and B$_6$; thiamin; niacin; fiber; riboflavin; folate; magnesium; potassium; and manganese. Boosts immune system; promotes healthy skin, eyes, heart, immune and nervous systems, and muscles; reduces inflammation and bone loss; regulates blood sugar

LEAN PROTEIN

Chicken   Vitamin B$_6$, selenium, and niacin. Reduces stress; promotes healthy skin, immune system, and heart

Eggs   Riboflavin and selenium. Strengthen immune system, prevent acne

Greek yogurt   vitamin B$_{12}$, potassium, zinc, riboflavin, and calcium. Increases energy; promotes healthy skin, hair, bones, muscles, and nervous system; prevents PMS; reduces stress; clears up acne

Lean beef   vitamins B$_6$ and B$_{12}$, zinc, and selenium. Reduces stress; promotes healthy skin, immune system, and hair

Salmon   Thiamin, riboflavin, niacin, vitamins B_6 and B_{12}, and selenium. Contains anti-aging properties, improves memory, strengthens immune system, prevents acne, increases energy, reduces stress

Shrimp   Niacin, vitamins B_{12} and D, iron, and selenium. Promotes healthy heart, skin, hair, bones, and muscles; boosts immunity

Tofu   Calcium, iron, magnesium, manganese, and selenium. Promotes strong bones and muscles; reduces inflammation

Turkey   Niacin and selenium. Promotes healthy heart, boosts immunity

HERBS AND SPICES

Basil   Vitamins E, C, K, and B_6; riboflavin; niacin; fiber; folate; calcium; iron; magnesium; phosphorus; potassium; zinc; and manganese. Contains anti-aging properties; balances hormones; strengthens immune system; prevents acne; increases metabolism; reduces stress; promotes healthy heart, muscles, and bones; reduces pain and inflammation; improves vision

Cilantro   Fiber; vitamins A, C, E, K, and B_6; riboflavin; niacin; folate; calcium; iron; magnesium; potassium; and manganese. Promotes healthy heart, skin, eyes, hair, immune and nervous systems, and muscles; reduces inflammation; increases energy; regulates blood sugar

Cinnamon   Vitamin K, iron, fiber, calcium, and manganese. Regulates blood sugar, promotes strong bones and heart, reduces inflammation

Cocoa   Potassium, zinc, fiber, iron, magnesium, and manganese. Reduces stress, inflammation, fatigue, and pain; promotes strong bones and muscles

Garlic   Calcium, selenium, vitamins C and B_6, and manganese. Boosts immunity, increases metabolism, reduces inflammation

Ginger   Vitamin C, magnesium, potassium, and manganese. Increases metabolism, reduces inflammation, promotes healthy bones and muscles

Mint   Niacin, phosphorus, zinc, fiber, vitamins A and C, riboflavin, folate, calcium, iron, magnesium, potassium, and manganese. Promotes a healthy heart, clears up acne, increases metabolism, strengthens immune system, reduces pain and inflammation

Parsley   Vitamins E, B_6, A, C, and K; thiamin; riboflavin; niacin; zinc; fiber; folate; calcium; iron; magnesium; potassium; and manganese. Contains anti-aging properties, balances hormones, promotes healthy heart, clears up acne and inflammation, boosts immune system

Rosemary   Vitamins B_6, A, and C; magnesium; potassium; fiber; folate; calcium; iron; and manganese. Reduces stress; promotes healthy skin, immune system, bones, muscles, heart

WHOLE GRAINS, NUTS, BEANS, AND SEEDS

Almonds   Magnesium, vitamin E, manganese, omega-3, and omega-6. Reduce pain, migraines, and inflammation; contain anti-aging properties; promote healthy skin, bones, and joints

Black beans   Thiamin, magnesium, manganese, fiber, and folate. Contain anti-aging properties; promote strong bones, heart, and muscles

Brown rice   Selenium and manganese. Boosts immunity, promotes healthy bones

Cashews   Magnesium and manganese. Reduce pain and migraines; promote strong bones and muscles and healthy nervous system

Chickpeas   Fiber, vitamin B$_6$, folate, and manganese. Promote healthy heart, skin, immune system, and muscles

Flaxseeds   Magnesium, iron, fiber, and calcium. Reduce pain, migraines, and fatigue; promote healthy muscles, heart, bones, and nervous system

Hemp seeds   Zinc, omega-3, and magnesium. Reduce fatigue, depression, and inflammation

Oats   Fiber, thiamin, magnesium, and manganese. Promote healthy heart and bones, contain anti-aging properties, improve memory

Peanuts   Omega-3 and omega-6, vitamin A, and calcium. Promote healthy skin; reduce depression, inflammation, pain, and symptoms of PMS

Pecans   Omega-3 and omega-6, vitamin A, and calcium. Promote healthy skin; reduce depression, inflammation, pain, and symptoms of PMS

Pine nuts   Omega-6 and calcium. Reduce inflammation and pain, promote strong bones

Quinoa   Magnesium and manganese. Reduces pain and migraines, promotes strong bones

Sesame seeds   Calcium, iron, magnesium, and manganese. Promote strong bones and muscles; reduce inflammation

Sunflower seeds   Thiamin, vitamin B$_6$, magnesium, manganese, and vitamin E. Contain anti-aging properties, improve memory, reduce stress and pain, promote healthy skin, balance hormones

Walnuts   Omega-3 and omega-6, calcium, iron, and vitamin B$_6$. Reduce depression, inflammation, pain, stress, and the symptoms of PMS; promote strong bones, healthy skin, strong immune system

HEALTHY FATS

Avocados   Fiber, vitamins K and C, folate, and potassium. Promote healthy heart, muscles, and bones; increase metabolism and energy; contain anti-aging properties

Coconuts   Reduce inflammation, pain, and symptoms of PMS

Olive oil   Omega-6 and iron. Reduces inflammation, pain, fatigue, and symptoms of PMS

Universal Conversion Chart

OVEN TEMPERATURE EQUIVALENTS

250°F = 120°C

275°F = 135°C

300°F = 150°C

325°F = 160°C

350°F = 180°C

375°F = 190°C

400°F = 200°C

425°F = 220°C

450°F = 230°C

475°F = 240°C

500°F = 260°C

MEASUREMENT EQUIVALENTS

Measurements should always be level unless directed otherwise.

⅛ teaspoon = 0.5 ml

¼ teaspoon = 1 ml

½ teaspoon = 2 ml

1 teaspoon = 5 ml

1 tablespoon = 3 teaspoons = ½ fluid ounce = 15 ml

2 tablespoons = ⅛ cup = 1 fluid ounce = 30 ml

4 tablespoons = ¼ cup = 2 fluid ounces = 60 ml

5⅓ tablespoons = ⅓ cup = 3 fluid ounces = 80 ml

8 tablespoons = ½ cup = 4 fluid ounces = 120 ml

10⅔ tablespoons = ⅔ cup = 5 fluid ounces = 160 ml

12 tablespoons = ¾ cup = 6 fluid ounces = 180 ml

16 tablespoons = 1 cup = 8 fluid ounces = 240 ml

Index

NOTE: Page references in *italics* indicate photographs.